FIBER FUELED RECIPE BOOK

Tasty And Easy Made Recipes To Optimize Your
Microbiome And For Rapid Weight Loss. Includes A
7-Days Meal Plan

Good and Healthy Academy

TABLE OF CONTENTS

INTRODUCTION

Dietary fiber (British spelling fibre) or roughage is the part of food that cannot be broken down by human digestive enzymes. **It has two Chief elements:**

Soluble Fiber – This is the fiber that dissolves in water. Fibers can be found as beta-glucans in barley, oats, mushrooms and uncooked guar gum. Psyllium is a viscous fiber. Psyllium is a fiber that keeps water as it goes through the gastrointestinal tract. Fiber is viscous and stays so long in the gastrointestinal tract that in people, it could lead to a sense of fullness. Exceptions are inulin (in onions), wheat dextrin, oligosaccharides, and resistant starches (in beans and peanuts), which can be nonviscous.

Insoluble Fiber – This is the fiber that doesn't dissolve in water. Examples are wheat bran, cellulose, and lignin. Ground insoluble fiber activates the secretion of mucus from the intestine, supplying bulking. Some sorts of fiber may be fermented in the colon. Dietary fiber consists of other polysaccharides plant components like cellulose, resistant starch, immune dextrins, inulin, lignins, chitins (in parasites), pectins, beta-glucans, and oligosaccharides. Some kinds of fiber absorb water to develop. Some insoluble kinds of fiber have bulking action and aren't fermented. An insoluble fiber supply containing a significant amount of lignin may change metabolism and the speed of fibers. Other kinds of insoluble fiber, especially resistant carbohydrates, are fermented to create short-chain fatty acids, which can be more active and confer health benefits. Health gain from dietary fiber and whole grains could include a decreased risk of passing and reduced levels of coronary heart disease, colon cancer, and type 2 diabetes. Food sources of dietary fiber have been split based on whether they provide fiber or not. Plant foods contain both kinds of fiber according to the features of fermentability and viscosity of the plant. The benefits of consuming fiber depend on which kind of fiber is absorbed and which advantages does is give to the digestive system. Bulking fibers -- like cellulose, hemicellulose, and psyllium absorb and hold water, promoting regularity. Fibers like psyllium and beta-glucan thicken the mass. Fermentable

2

fibers like resistant starch and inulin feed the germs and microbiota of the intestine, and are summoned to produce short-chain fatty acids, which have varied roles in gastrointestinal health.

CHAPTER 1
SCFA (SHORT CHAIN FATTY ACIDS)

Short-Chain Fatty Acid

Short-chain fatty acids (SCFAs) are fatty acids with fewer than six electrons. Aside from intestinal microbial fermentation of indigestible foods, SCFAs are the primary energy source of colonocytes, which makes them critical to gastrointestinal health.

Functions

When fiber is fermented, SCFAs are produced in the colon. Macronutrient composition (carbohydrate, protein, or fat) of diets influences circulating SCFAs. Acetate, propionate, and butyrate are the three most frequent SCFAs. SCFAs and medium-chain fatty acids are mainly absorbed via the portal vein through lipid digestion, whereas long-chain fatty acids have been packaged into chylomicrons, enter lymphatic capillaries, and then move to the bloodstream in the subclavian vein. SCFAs have varied functions in the body. They could impact the creation of energy, lipids, and vitamins. They are also able to affect appetite and cardiometabolic health. Butyrate is especially essential for colon health since it is the principal energy supply for colonocytes. The liver may utilize acetate for vitality.

The Way Short-Chain Fatty Acids Affect Health And Weight

Short-chain fatty acids are made by the favorable Germs in the gut. They are the chief source of nourishment for those cells on your colon. Short-chain fatty acids can also play a significant part in disease and health. They may lessen the possibility of inflammatory diseases, type 2 diabetes, obesity, cardiovascular disease, and other problems.

What Exactly Are Short-Chain Fatty Acids?

Short-chain fatty acids are fatty acids with over 6 Carbon (C) atoms. They're created if the friendly gut bacteria ferment fiber into your colon, and also, therefore, are the primary source of energy for the cells lining your colon. Because of this, they play a significant role in colon health. Excessive fatty acids have been utilized for different purposes within the body. By way of instance, they can provide approximately 10 percent of your daily caloric requirements. Short-chain fatty acids are also involved in the metabolism of all nutrients such as carbohydrates and fat.

About 95 percent of the Short-chain fatty acids in the human body are:

- Acetate (C2)

- Propionate (C3)

- Butyrate (C4)

Propionate is involved in generating glucose for the Liver, whereas acetate and butyrate are integrated into other fatty acids and cholesterol. Several things impact the quantity of short-chain fatty acids on your colon, such as how many germs are found, the food supply, and also the time it takes food to travel through your digestive tract.

Food Resources Of Short-Chain Fatty Acids

Eating lots of fiber-rich foods, like fruits, vegetables, and beans, is connected to a growth in short-chain fatty acids. An analysis of 153 people found positive relationships between a greater ingestion of plant foods and raised amounts of short-chain fatty acids in feces. On the other hand, the quantity and type of fiber you eat influences the makeup of bacteria in your gut, which influences what short-chain fatty acids are created. As an instance, various studies have proven that eating more fiber raises butyrate production, while reducing your fiber consumption reduces generation.

The next types of fiber would be best for its creation of short-chain fatty acids in the colon:

- **Inulin:** you can get inulin from artichokes, garlic, leeks, onions, wheat, rye, and asparagus.

- **Fructooligosaccharides (FOS):** FOS can be found in a variety of fruits and vegetables, such as carrots, onions, garlic, and asparagus.

- **Resistant starch:** you'll be able to get resistant starch from potatoes, barley, rice, legumes, green peas, legumes, and potatoes which were cooked and then chilled.

- **Pectin:** Great sources of pectin include apples, pears, apricots, oranges, carrots, and many others.

- **Arabinoxylan:** Arabinoxylan is located in cereal grains. It is by far the most frequent fiber in wheat germ.

- **Guar gum:** Guar gum may be extracted from guar beans that are beans.

- Some Kinds of butter, cheese, and cow's milk comprise Small quantities of butyrate.

Short-Chain Fatty Acids and Digestive Disorders

Fatty acids might be beneficial for treating some gastrointestinal ailments. By way of instance, butyrate has positive effects on the gut.

Diarrhea

Your gut bacteria convert pectin and starch into Short-Chain Fatty Acids. Ingesting them, and acids have been demonstrated to decrease diarrhea.

Inflammatory Bowel Disease

Crohn's disease and ulcerative colitis are the two primary Kinds of inflammatory bowel disease (IBD). Both are characterized by bowel inflammation. Due to its properties, butyrate was used to deal with these conditions both. Studies in mice have demonstrated that butyrate supplements decrease gut inflammation, and acetate supplements had comparable advantages. Lower degrees of fatty acids have been connected to worsened esophageal disorders. Human studies indicate that fatty acids can improve symptoms of Crohn's disease and ulcerative colitis. Research involving 22 patients with ulcerative colitis discovered that symptoms were improved by consuming 60 g of oat bran every day. Another study found that supplements resulted in 53 percent of Crohn's disease sufferers in enhancements and remission. For ulcerative colitis patients, an enema of all fatty acids helped reduce symptoms.

Short-Chain Fatty Acids and Oral Cancer

Fatty acids can play an Integral role in Prevention and therapy of cancers such as colon cancer. Laboratory studies show that butyrate prevents the development of tumor cells; helps maintain colon cells healthy, and promotes cancer cell destruction from the colon. The mechanics behind this isn't well-understood. Observational studies indicate a connection between high-fiber diets and a decreased risk of colon cancer. Experts suggest that the creation of fatty acids might be responsible for it. In a study, the mice who didn't possess the germs, obtained not tumors than mice onto a diet, whose bowels contained bacteria. Interestingly, the diet alone -- with no germs didn't have protective effects against colon cancer. A low-fiber diet -- despite all the butyrate-producing germs -- was likewise ineffective. This implies that the advantages exist if there is a diet combined with the bacteria in the intestine. Human studies offer mixed results. Some suggest a link between cancer risk and high-fiber diets, but others find no connection. Nevertheless, those studies did not appear in the gut bacteria, and differences in gut bacteria can play a role.

Short-Chain Fatty Acids and Diabetes

An overview of the signs reported that butyrate could have Positive effects with type 2 diabetes in animals and people. The review also emphasized that there is apparently an imbalance in gut germs in people with diabetes. Fatty acids have been proven to improve activity in the muscle and liver tissues. In animal research, blood glucose levels improved in rats and diabetic mice. However, there are studies and the results have been combined. A study found that propionate supplements decreased blood glucose levels, but another study found that short-chain fatty acid supplements didn't significantly affect blood glucose control in healthy men and women. A number of studies also have reported relationships between fiber and also blood glucose control and insulin sensitivity. Yet this result is usually seen in those that are overweight or insulin-resistant, rather than in people.

Short-Chain Fatty Acids and Weight Reduction

The makeup of bacteria in the gut could impact Absorption and energy regulation. Various studies have revealed that fatty acids regulate metabolism by reducing fat storage and increasing fat burning. The number of fatty acids in the bloodstream is decreased while this happens, and it might help protect against weight gain.

This result has been analyzed by animal studies. Following a 5-week therapy, butyrate obese mice dropped 10.2 percent of their initial body fat, and body fat has been decreased by 10 percent. In rats, storage was decreased by acetate supplements. The evidence linking fatty acids is based on test-tube and animal studies.

Short-Chain Fatty Acids and Heart Health

Diets have been connected by observational studies to a reduced risk of cardiovascular disease. On the other hand, the association's potency is based upon the source and the fiber type. In people, fiber consumption has been linked to inflammation. Some reason fiber reduces cardiovascular disease risk might be due to the creation of fatty acids. Studies in people and animals have reported that cholesterol levels were decreased by fatty acids. Butyrate is considered to interact with genes, which make cholesterol thereby reducing cholesterol generation. By way of instance, cholesterol generation decreased from the livers of rats given nutritional supplements that were propionate. Cholesterol levels were decreased by acetic acid. As the quantity of cholesterol diminished from the bloodstream, the result was found in humans.

CHAPTER 2
CONS OF CRAP AND UNHEALTHY FOODS ON HEALTH

Junk Food

Junk food is Sugar or fat, with little dietary fiber, protein, vitamins, nutritional supplements, or other kinds of value. Definitions vary from purpose and above time. Some foods, such as meat ready with fat, might be regarded as junk food. The expression of HFSS foods (high in fat, sugar, and salt) can be used synonymously. Although foods can't be described as crap food, fast food restaurants, and fast food tend to be equated with crap food. Junk food is foods that are highly processed. Concerns about the health consequences caused by a crap food-heavy diet have led to public health awareness campaigns and limitations on purchase and advertising.

Source of the Term

The term junk food dates back to the 1950s, although its coinage was imputed to Michael F. Jacobson of the Center for Science in the Public Interest, in 1972. Back in 1952, the term appeared in a headline at the Lima, Ohio, News," 'Junk Foods' Cause Serious Malnutrition", within a reprint of a 1948 article from the Ogden, Utah, Standard-Examiner, initially titled," Dr. Brady's Health Column: More Junk Than Food". From the report, Dr. Brady writes, "What Mrs. H calls 'crap' I predict cheat meals. That's or processed sugar syrup and anything made of bread. By way of instance, white bread, crackers, cake, candies, ice cream soda, chocolate malted, sundaes, sweetened carbonated drinks "The word stuffing meals could be traced back to 1916 into paper cites.

Definitions

In Andrew F. Smith's Encyclopedia of Quick and Junk Food, crap food is described as "those business goods, such as candy, bakery products, ice cream, salty snacks and soft beverages, that have little if any nutritional value but has lots of salt, calories, and carbs. Many are while not all of foods are junk foods. Fast foods have been foods

14

served after ordering. Some quick foods are high in carbs and low in nutritional value, while some other fast foods, like salads, might be reduced in carbs and high in nutritional value." Junk food offers calories, providing small or none of the protein, vitamins, minerals, or minerals necessary for a diet. Many foods, like tacos, pizza, and hamburgers, may be thought of as junk foods or healthy, based on their ingredients and preparation procedures. Things fall such as breakfast cereals which are flour or corn and higher fructose corn syrup or sugar. The bureau for its UK ad business, the United Kingdom's Advertising Standards Authority, utilizes. Foods are scored for "nutrition (energy, saturated fat, full sugar and sodium) anodic" nutrition (fruit, vegetables and nut material, protein and fiber). The distinction between C and A scores decides if a food or drink is categorized as HFSS (high in fat, sugar, and salt; a word synonymous with crap food). As meaningless, the crap food tag is described in Panic Country: Unpicking the Myths we are Told about Health and Food: food is food, and then it is not a crap when there is value. Co-editor Vincent Marks explains, "To label a food as 'crap' is another way of saying, 'I disapprove it' There are bad foods - which is, poor mixtures and amounts of food - however, there aren't any 'bad foods' except the ones that are very bad through pollution or corrosion."

History

According to an article at the New York Times, "Let Us Now Praise the excellent Men of Steak", "The history of crap food is a mostly American narrative: It's existed for centuries, in many regions of the earth, but nobody has ever done a much better job inventing numerous forms of it, branding it, even mass-producing it, making people wealthy it off and, of course, eating it" Cracker Jack, the confection, is credited as the popular name brand crap food; it enrolled in 1896 was made in Chicago, and became the most popular candy in the world.

Popularity and Allure

Waste food in its different forms and also a part of contemporary culture. In the United States, yearly fast-food sales are in the region of $160 billion, in contrast to grocery sales of $620 billion (a figure that also has junk food in the shape of convenience meals, snack foods, and candies). Back in 1976, the united states Top 10 pop tune,

"Junk Food Junkie", clarified a junk food enthusiast who dared to stick to a wholesome diet daily, while at night gorges on Hostess Twinkies and Fritos corn chips, McDonald's and KFC. Thirty-six decades later, Time put the Twinkie at #1 in a post titled, "Best 10 Iconic Junk Foods": "Not merely...a mainstay on the supermarket shelves and in our bellies, they have been a staple in our culture and, most importantly, in our hearts. Often criticized for its absence of any nutritional value at all, the Twinkie has been able to act as a cultural and gastronomical icon" America envisions on July 21. Origins are uncertain; it's one of about 175 US food and beverage days, most generated by "individuals who wish to market more food", occasionally aided by elected officials at the request of a trade association or product category. "In honor of this day," Time in 2014 released, "5 Crazy Junk Food Combinations". Headlines from other local and national media policy include: "Celebrate National Waste Food Day with... Beer-Flavored Oreos?" (MTV); "National Junk Food Day: Pick your favorite carbonated treats in this survey" (Baltimore); "Stars' favorite junk food" (Los Angeles); "A Nutritionist's Guide to National Junk Food Day" with "Presents for

Splurging" (Huffington Post); and "It Is National Junk Food Day: obtained snacks?" (Kansas City).As for crap food's allure, there's not any definitive scientific response; both bodily and psychological variables are mentioned. Food makers spend billions of dollars on development and research to make flavor profiles that activate the affinity for fat, salt, and sugar. Consumption ends in pleasurable; addictive that is probable, effects in the mind. At precisely the exact same time marketing campaigns are deployed; the taste will be trumped by producing brand loyalties that research has shown. The explanations for this aren't apparent; although it's well-established more junk food is eaten by the poor than the affluent. Few studies have focused on variations in meal perception based on socioeconomic standing (SES); a few types of research which have discerned according to SES imply that the effectively challenged do not perceive wholesome food considerably differently than every other section of the populace. A recent study into scarcity, combining behavioral science and economics, indicates that confronted with intense financial instability, where the next meal might not be a positive thing, judgment is impaired and the drive would be to the instantaneous satisfaction of crap food, rather than to creating the essential investment from the longer-term advantages of a healthy diet.

Health Effects

If junk food is absorbed often, the surplus fat, Simple Carbs, and sugars produce cardiovascular disease, risk of obesity, and other chronic health conditions. A case study on the consumption of foods in Ghana indicated A correlation between consumption. The Report claims that obesity led to complex health issues that are associated with such Upsurge of heart attack cases. Studies show that as early as the age of 30, Arteries lay the groundwork for potential heart attacks and could start flushing. Consumers tend to eat a lot in one sitting Satisfied their desire with crap food are not as inclined to consume foods Such as fruit or vegetables. Effects have been suggested by testing on rats of Crap food which may manifest in people. A Scripps Research Institute Research in 2008 indicated that brain activity alters in a manner very similar to drugs such as heroin and cocaine. After many weeks With access to junk food, rat brains' pleasure centers became Desensitized, requiring meals for enjoyment Off and replaced with a wholesome diet, the rats starved for a couple of weeks Nutritious fare of eating. A 2007 study from the British Journal Found that rats who eat crap food improved the Probability of eating habits. Additional research has been performed on health in people on sugary foods' effect, and has suggested that energy levels can be negatively impacted by the consumption of junk food and Psychological well-being. In a study Nutrition of 57 foods/drinks of 4000 kids at Four and a half years have been gathered from the report. At age seven, 4000 kids were awarded the Strengths and Difficulties Questionnaire (SDQ), Psychological, with five scales: hyperactivity, conduct issues, peer problems Symptoms, and behavior. A one standard deviation rise in crap Food was linked in 33 percent of those subjects to hyperactivity that was excess Junk food being consumed by To the end that children at age seven Are more inclined to be at the upper third of their scale that is hyperactivity. There wasn't any significant correlation between junk food along with the other scales.

10 Motives Junk Food Is Bad For Your Health

Over the Last Few decade's samosas Etc, pizzas, hamburgers, rolls Frankies fries have penetrated every corner of our nation. You step out of your residence and you're going to find them being served from roadside corners and restaurants into college and office canteens. But have you ever wondered why are they known as 'crap'? The term 'crap' describes something useless and extra. And of your delicious foods do justice. The results this crap food has on your health are dreadful, no matter if you've got them once every so often, double in a week or two daily. Have a peek at this crap plays a role.

- **Junk food might be the reason for your tiredness:** Though junk food and fast food makes you feel full and satisfied, they lack all the necessary nutrients such as carbohydrates and proteins to help keep your body healthy and energized. If you eat junk food each time you are hungry, then you might feel chronically exhausted. It may reduce your energy levels that it might become hard for you to execute your activities.

- **Junks food can cause depression in teens:** a great deal of hormonal changes occurs in teens making them vulnerable to mood swings and behavioral alterations. And a wholesome diet plays an essential part in keeping that equilibrium that is hormonal. 58 percent increases the probability of teens because junk food deficiency those nutrients.

- **It impairs digestion:** those people that are hooked on fatty junk foods are certain to have digestive issues such as gastroesophageal reflux disorder (GERD) and irritable bowel syndrome (IBS). That is because junk food is fried. The petroleum in the crap food gets hauled in the gut resulting in. They cause irritation of the gut lining since they're too hot, and they also lack the fiber that's essential for good digestion.

- **It causes changes in blood glucose levels**: Junk food is full of processed sugar that sets your metabolism under pressure. Processed sugar causes the pancreas to secrete more quantity of insulin to stop a drastic spike in your glucose levels. After you consume, since junk food lacks levels of carbs and fats, the degree of blood glucose fall. This makes you feel raises you craving to get crap food.

- **It impacts the brain functioning:** A study published in the journal Brain, Behavior, and Immunity indicates that one week of eating crap food is sufficient to activate memory impairment in rats. A recent study indicates that poor fats (Tran's fats) from junk foods will substitute healthful fats from the brain and interferes with its normal signaling mechanism. Studies in animals also have demonstrated that the capacity slows down.

- **It raises the chance of coronary disease:** Junks food raises cholesterol and cholesterol levels that are significant risk factors for the development of heart ailments. Moreover, the time is accumulated over by fats out of crap food within your own body. The more weight you wear, the greater your risk of experiencing heart attacks.

- **It can lead to kidney disorder:** The reason you

cannot say no to chips is because they contain a high number of finely processed sodium that raises salivation and secretion of enzymes which enriches your cravings. The number of fats and affects the gut function also sodium from sodium raises blood pressure.

- **It can harm your liver** elevated levels of trans fats found in many junk foods can lead to deposition of fats from the liver, which may lead to liver dysfunction.

- **It can lead to type 2 diabetes** when you consume a wholesome diet, your body gets a steady supply of sugar which helps to keep insulin sensitivity. However, while you eat only junk foods, the surplus stress exerted onto your metabolism may influence the ability of the human body to use insulin correctly.

- **It raises your chance of cancer** study published in the European Journal of Cancer Prevention demonstrated that consuming a lot of fast foods that are high in fat and sugar may improve your likelihood of developing pancreatic cancer. Another study by the Fred Hutchinson Cancer Research Center, Seattle revealed that men who ate foods over double had an increased probability of prostate cancer.

Harmful Effects of Junk Food

Crap foods' dim side isn't an unknown truth. Several research studies have revealed that processed foods have significantly worsened other chronic ailments, cardiovascular disease and diabetes, and childhood obesity. Recently, the Delhi Government required a crackdown on junk food that's offered in schools and over 50 meters of these. Not only do they add inches to your waist, but scientists and scientists also have suggested through different research that junk food may actually cause considerable harm to your mind. The worrying bit is that it is not merely years of bad eating, but normal use of junk food for a few days may cause a psychological meltdown. The more junk food you eat, the not as likely you should eat the nutrients your body depends upon. You are aware that junk food may damage your health, but you could have understood the effects of junk food on how your mind works.

It Can Lead To Learning and Memory Issues

An analysis published in the American Journal of Clinical Nutrition Nutrition in 2011 revealed that healthy men and women who ate junk food for just 5 times played poorly on cognitive tests that measured attention, rate, and disposition. It reasoned that your memory can be frequently deteriorated by eating crap food for five days. This likely originates from the fact that a bad or poisonous diet may cause specific chemical reactions that result in inflammation in the hippocampus region of the brain that's related to memory and particular recognition. Foods that are high in fat and sugar may suppress the action of a mind peptide named BDNF (brain-derived neurotrophic factor) which assists with learning and memory formation. In addition, the mind comprises synapses that are responsible for memory and learning. Eating too many calories may interfere with functioning and the production of all those synapses.

Increases the Risk of Dementia

It has been one of the scariest discoveries with the use of junk foods. You will know that insulin is produced in the pancreas and assists in the transport of sugar to fuel the human body. Insulin is generated in the mind in which it aids in forming memories and carrying signals between nerve cells. A study conducted in the Brown University demonstrates that too much fatty foods and sweets can considerably boost the insulin levels in our body. The same as in the case of Type 2 Diabetes, together with high amounts of insulin, the mind stops responding to the hormone and become immune to it. This can limit our capacity to think, remember, or develop memories, thereby increasing the chance of dementia. Chemical Suzanne de la Monte, M.D., a professor of pathology, neurology, and neurosurgery at Rhode Island Hospital and the Alpert Medical School of Brown University was the first to discover this institution. After this discovery, most scientists refer to Alzheimer's because of a kind of diabetes of their mind.

Lessens Its Capability to Control Hunger

Consumption of fats found in fried and processed foods may send mixed signals to the mind that makes it hard to process what you've consumed and how hungry will be. This is why you wind up overeating. Brain acts demand a dose of essential fatty acids such as omega-3 and omega-6. Deficiency of both of these components raises the possibility of other issues and attention deficit disorder, arthritis, and dementia disease. Overconsumption of junk foods can displace those with Tran's fats that are more difficult to digest. A 2011 research demonstrates that Trans fats can lead to inflammation in the hypothalamus, the portion of the mind that comprising neurons to control body fat. In worst situations, the practice of overeating may be comparable to drug dependency to an extent which emphasizing junk foods can activate the pleasure centers of the mind greater than getting medication.

It Can Because of Chemical Changes Which May Lead To Depression

A Good Deal of research shows that foods high in glucose and fat changes the action of the mind which makes it reliant on foods. A study conducted in the University of Montreal on mice revealed they endured with withdrawal symptoms following their routine junk food diet has been discontinued. In people, these withdrawal symptoms may result in the inability to handle stress, because you feel miserable and you would return to these foods to comfort yourself and manage those feelings. You might be caught in a vicious cycle before it is known by you. By consuming an excessive amount of fast food that you may miss out on essential nutrients such as amino acid tryptophan, feelings of depression may increase. An imbalance of fatty acids is just another reason.

This Makes You Impatient and Can Cause Uncontrollable Cravings

Eating doughnut or a cupcake may spike your blood glucose levels allow you to feel happy and fulfilled but when they return to ordinary you're left feeling even more irritable. Food is stuffed with carbohydrates that cause your blood sugar levels to fluctuate. It can lead to tiredness, confusion, and stress if your glucose levels dip to a degree. With high levels of sugars and carbohydrates, you typically eat too quickly and too much to fulfill your cravings. Whilst dealing with things, this may inculcate an impatient behavior. Quick foods and processed foods might be sprinkled with synthetic flavorings and additives such as sodium benzoate that will boost hyperactivity Quick foods are specially made to be addictive in character with elevated levels of salts, sugars, and carbohydrates that make you crave them. The addictive nature of fast food can make your mind crave them even if you aren't hungry.

CHAPTER 3
ADVANTAGES OF FIBERS FOR WELLNESS AND WEIGHT LOSS

What's Fiber?

Many People associate fiber together with physiological and health Functions we would rather not consider. Eating foods high in fiber may do more than keep you regular. It may decrease your risk for heart disease, stroke, obesity, and diabetes, enhance the health of the skin, and also help you shed weight. It could help prevent colon cancer. Fiber, also referred to as roughage, is the section of plant-based foods (fruits, grains, vegetables, nuts, and legumes) the body cannot break down. It moves to flush down cholesterol and damaging toxins from the human body, easing bowel motions, and maintaining your tract fit and clean.

Fiber comes in 2 Varieties: Magnesium and Magnesium.

- Insoluble fiber doesn't dissolve in water. It's the fiber that helps to reduce constipation and can be found in whole grains, wheat cereals, and vegetables like celery, carrots, and tomatoes.

- Soluble fiber dissolves in water also helps decrease cholesterol and control glucose levels. Sources include nuts, oatmeal, beans, barley, and fruits like pears, berries, citrus fruits, and apples.

Many foods contain both insoluble and soluble fiber. In general, the organic and unprocessed the food, the greater it's in fiber. There's not any fiber in sugar, milk, or meat levels. Processed or "white" foods, like white bread, white rice, and pastries, have had all or most of their fiber eliminated.

Fiber In Fast Food

Fast food is usually convenient and cheap, but finding a Healthy meal with sufficient fiber can be a challenge. Many fast-food meals are packed with carbs, sodium, and fat with little or no dietary fiber. A seemingly healthy salad from a quick food restaurant can be light on fiber-- simple lettuce greens provide only about 0.5 grams of fiber per cup. Look for salads that have other vegetables, and whenever possible, up the fiber content by adding your own nuts, beans, or corn.

Other tips for getting more fiber from meals at fast-food restaurants:

- Choose sandwiches, burgers, or subs which include a whole wheat bun or whole grain bread.

- Try a veggie burger. Many taste far better than they used to and contain a couple of times more fiber than a meat burger.

- Pick a side of beans to get a wholesome fiber boost.

- Pick a salad fries or potato chips.

- Combining a baked potato and a side of bread, available at some burger chains, may make a yummy, high-fiber meal.

- Many chains provide oatmeal bowls for breakfast, a greater fiber choice than many breakfast sandwiches. Try to choose lower sugar variations if possible.

- End a fast food meal with a fruit cup, fruit and yogurt parfait, apple pieces, or a bit of fruit.

Fiber Supplements

While the best way to get fiber in your daily diet is from foods naturally rich in fiber--fruit, vegetables, whole grains, legumes, nuts--if that proves difficult, taking a fiber supplement will make up the shortfall. Supplements may also be useful to accelerate your daily fiber consumption as you transition to a high-fiber diet plan. Fiber supplements come in many different forms, including powders you dissolve in water or add to food, chewable tablets, and wafers. But, there are some drawbacks to getting your fiber from nutritional supplements instead of foods that are salty:

- Fiber supplements won't supply the very same vitamins, minerals, and other nutrients offered by high-quality foods.

- Supplements help you manage your weight or will not fill up you.

- Fiber supplements may interact with some drugs, including the drug warfarin medications, and certain antidepressants. Check with your physician before taking a fiber supplement, or pharmacist about potential drug interactions.

- In case you have diabetes, fiber supplements can reduce your glucose levels so again, check with your healthcare provider before adding supplements to your daily diet plan.

- If you decide to take a fiber supplement, begin with small Drink lots of fluids, and amounts and slowly build-up to prevent any bloating and gas.

Is Fiber The Essential Ingredient To Weight Loss?

A few Years Back, it had been the f-word that nobody wanted to use. It's plastered all around packages at the grocery store and hailed from nutritionists as a few one nutrient. The f-word is an individual's fiber, and it's time to discuss fiber for weight reduction. Studies peg foods full of fiber to a reduced risk of cardiovascular disease, diabetes, and cancer and that fiber for weight loss might be the crucial ingredient to losing weight without feeling hungry. For example, researchers at Harvard Medical School found that women who increased their consumption of high-fiber or whole-grain foods over a 12-year period were half as likely to become obese as those who decreased their consumption. (P.S. Here is the difference between whole wheat and whole grain)

So How Does Fiber Work, Anyway?

It's the part of plant foods--vegetables, fruits, Nuts beans, legumes, and seeds --that your body can not digest. There are two types of fiber: insoluble, which aids food pass and potassium, which can help remove fat and lower cholesterol. Due to sugars, soluble fiber and fats enter your blood at a speed that is slower, giving a steady source of energy to you. "When you consume foods that lack fiber, your blood glucose may spike quickly. Then it crashes, resulting in hunger and overeating," says Tanya Zuckerbrot, R.D., writer of The F-Factor Diet. The fiber of food has the better. "Fiber-packed goods tend to be low-cal, so you can consume a lot," states Zuckerbrot. "Fiber makes you full, since it swells in your gut when it absorbs fluid." Fiber is also a heart enthusiast: It will help to lower cholesterol and blood pressure, and it increases blood circulation. The effect on cholesterol of soluble fiber is so potent that the FDA allows organizations to promote this fact on goods such as oatmeal. The nutrient can also reduce amounts of C-reactive protein (CRP), a marker for inflammation, which has been associated with cardiovascular disease, diabetes, and cancer. In a study people with the highest fiber intake had been 63 percent less likely to have elevated levels of CRP than people who followed diets that are lower-fiber.

Why You Need More Fiber for Weight Loss (And In General)

Most people (latest reports quote about 95% of Americans) aren't getting sufficient fiber. The average woman absorbs about 10 to 15 grams of fiber per day-- about half of what is required to meet with the recommendation of 25 g. And experts say that more is much better--about 30 to 40 grams a day, according to David L. Katz, M.D., M.P.H., an associate professor adjunct of public health and director of the Prevention Research Center at Yale University School of Medicine. But before you put that healthy-looking loaf of bread in your shopping cart, make sure to understand what you're getting, advises Kathy McManus, R.D., director of nutrition at Brigham and Women's Hospital in Boston. Read the label carefully and check the fiber content. Start looking for at least 3 g of fiber daily in bread and decide on a cereal. Other label buzzwords to watch for:

- **"Whole"**: as in"100 percent whole wheat" or "whole-grain oats." The primary ingredient listed should be a whole grain.

- **"Great source of fiber"**: This indicates you're getting at least 5 grams of fiber in each serving, while "good source" implies that one serving contains at least 2.5 g of fiber.

- **"Graham flour"**: A type of whole wheat germ. Yes, it's whole grain. But remember to check the fiber material.

- **"Whole-grain meals"**: Each serving has to include at least 51 percent whole grains. However, depending on the item, the quantity of fiber might below. Breads contain more water than carbohydrates perform, so even if they are whole-grain, they will not necessarily contain fiber. Check the label.

- **"Made with whole grains"**: If the grains in question look far down on the components list, set the item back on the shelf.

- "**Multigrain**": The food is created with over one type of grain, but not necessarily whole grains. Check the fiber content as well as the ingredients list.

- **"100 percent wheat"**: When it doesn't say "whole," it is refined bread, so all of the fiber and nutrients were stripped off in processing.

- **"Enriched"**: This term indicates that some of the vitamins are added back after processing but the fiber hasn't. Skip it. (Asking for a friend, fine, me...Is it feasible to eat a lot of fiber?)

The 7-Day No-Hunger Fiber For Weight Loss Diet

Whether your goal is fiber for intestine for weight loss or fiber Health, eating a lot of this f-stuff is vital. If your diet is low in fiber (which means you do not eat a lot of fruits, veggies, legumes, nuts, and whole grains), then begin by adding one or two of the choices below each day, says Martha Gooldy Garcia, R.D., a dietitian in Fort Collins, Colorado who produced this eating plan for Shape. Should you experience any unpleasant side effects, like gas or bloating, let your body adapt before adding more. "Be sure to drink loads of water and stay active," suggests Garcia.

Fiber For Weight Loss Day 1

- **Breakfast:** Eat a bowl of cereal that is grated.

- **Lunch:** Add fruit, such as kiwi, cherries, or dried figs, to a salad.

- **Snack:** Munch on popcorn rather than potato chips.

- **Dinner:** Toss sliced peppers and diced broccoli into your skillet.

Fiber For Weight Loss Day 2

- Breakfast: Make toast with whole wheat bread rather than white.

- Lunch: Change your taco for a bean burrito.

- Snack: Whip up trail mix using high-quality cereal, nuts, and dried fruit.

- Dinner: place the peeler away--mashed potatoes taste good with the skins on.

Fiber For Weight Loss Day 3

- **Breakfast:** Consume a blueberry bran muffin instead of a bagel. (Or try one of these wholesome bagel hacks.)

- **Steak:** Eat brown rice with your Chinese takeout.

- **Snack:** Dip baby carrots and snap peas in hummus.

- **Dinner:** Utilize barley to create "pasta" salad.

Fiber For Weight Loss Day 4

- **Breakfast:** Make oatmeal with cinnamon, raisins, brown sugar, and skim milk.

- **Steak:** Try a wrap with a whole wheat tortilla rather than your usual sandwich.

- **Snack:** Order a new or frozen fruit smoothie.

- **Dinner:** Stir canned pumpkin to your favorite vegetable stew recipe.

Fiber For Weight Loss Day 5

- **Breakfast:** throw a couple of blueberries on your cereal.

- **Lunch:** Put black beans or chickpeas on your salad.

- **Snack:** Dip lentil chips into bean dip.

- **Dinner:** Make soup. Cook broccoli in poultry puree, and broth until tender.

Fiber For Weight Loss Day 6

- **Breakfast:** Sit back to whole wheat frozen waffles (or one of these healthy homemade waffle recipes).

- **Steak:** Rather than pepperoni pizza, have a whole wheat veggie piece.

- **Snack:** Nosh on apple slices topped with almond butter.

- **Dinner:** Serve a stir-fry with soba noodles (they're made with buckwheat).

Fiber For Weight Loss Day 7

- **Breakfast:** scatter the juice and eat an orange with your morning meal.

- **Lunch:** Fill on minestrone, lentil, or split-pea soup.

- **Snack:** Top whole-grain crackers with salsa.

- **Dinner:** rather than rice, try quinoa, a nutty-tasting, high-quality grain.

Easy Fiber For Weight Loss Swaps

Beneath, a few bonus hints for simple ways to increase your fiber intake at every meal of the day

- Instead of 1 cup apple juice (0.2 g fiber), attempt 1 apple (3.3 g fiber)

- Instead of 1 cup spaghetti (2.4 g fiber), try 1 cup whole-wheat spaghetti (6.3 g fiber)

- Instead of 1 cup long-grain white rice (0.6 g fiber), attempt 1 cup long-grain brown rice (3.5 g fiber)

- Instead of 1 cup instant mashed potatoes (1.7g fiber), attempt 1 baked sweet potato with skin (4.8g fiber)

- Instead of 1 cup macaroni (1.8 g fiber), try 1 cup barley (6 grams fiber)

- Instead of 1 cup peeled cucumber (0.8 g fiber), attempt 1 medium artichoke (3 g fiber)

- Instead of 1 cup iceberg lettuce (0.7 g fiber), attempt 1 cup romaine lettuce (1.2 g fiber)

- Instead of 1 slice white bread (0.6 g fiber, then attempt 1 slice hearty whole-wheat bread (3 g fiber)

- Rather than 1 oz potato chips (1.4 g fiber), try 3 cups air-popped popcorn (3.5 g fiber)

- Instead of a 1.55-ounce milk-chocolate bar (1.5 g fiber), attempt a 1.3-ounce whole-bean chocolate bar (6 grams fiber)

- Rather than 1 fig-bar cookie (0.7 g fiber), attempt 1 cup raspberries (8 g fiber)

CHAPTER 4
SOURCES OF FIBER TO DIETS
(FRUITS AND VEGETABLES)

How Much Fiber Do You Want Every Day?

The recommended daily fiber consumption is 28 grams, with Variations based on age and sex. Most Americans consume only about 16 g every day. The truth is: Less than 5 percent of Americans get enough daily fiber. If you do not eat enough fiber, what can you expect? In the short-term, you might sometimes feel constipated and sluggish. But a diet low in fiber may increase your risk for type 2 diabetes, such as cardiovascular disease and more serious problems. In case you have any concerns, reach out to your health care provider. A diet that includes lots of plant foods is the best way to get all the nutrients your body needs to function at its best, such as fiber. But that is not possible with our busy, demanding schedules. Fiber supplements such as Metamucil will help increase your everyday fiber intake. One serving of Metamucil's Sugar-Free and Real Sugar

Powders give you 3 g of dietary fiber per serving. New Metamucil users should start with one serving per day, and gradually increase to desired daily consumption.

High Fiber Foods To Add To Your Diet

You could be eating high fiber meals daily. Or you May find that some foods that you eat have fiber meal choices. If you're reaching the 28 grams of daily fiber intake, every 19, however, do you know? This food manual can help you determine how much fiber you're getting. Taking Metamucil daily can help make certain you get the recommended amount of fiber together with the foods that you enhance your diet plan.

Vegetables

Broccoli Flowerets

It requires about 9 cups of broccoli flowerets to reach the Daily recommended fiber consumption. High in sulforaphane, broccoli additionally adds 3.2 grams of fiber per cup. And it's low in calories, so add an additional helping of broccoli to help reach your fiber goals.

Brussels sprouts

These cabbages can be broiled, boiled, pan-fried, or Slaw sprouts. With 4 grams of fiber per cup, it requires approximately 7 cups of brussels sprouts to reach the fiber intake that is daily.

Asparagus

Have you noticed 83 spears on a single plate? Probably not, unless it's a meal. That is just how many asparagus spears it takes to hit the 28 grams of fiber. As an alternative to steamed asparagus attempt adding sliced asparagus spears to sandwiches or salads for a sweet, crispy taste.

Artichokes

Artichokes taste good on pizza Yummy vegetable steamed to perfection, or dip. But can you consume 4 artichokes in a day?

Acorn squash

Only cut the stem out, scoop the seeds and bake till Tender. Or prepare stuffed acorn squash using ground beef, quinoa, or wild rice. You'll want to eat about 3 cups of acorn squash to attain your fiber objectives.

Green peas

To larger, help with 9 grams of fiber per cup Helpings to add more fiber into your daily diet. You're going to need about 3 cups of peas to get the daily recommended fiber intake. Flavorful and healthy, green peas are a great source of iron, manganese, and vitamins A and C.

Turnip greens

A Superb source of beta carotene and vitamin turnip, K Greens possess a taste that is mild. They mixed to green smoothies, can be used like spinach and other greens, or juiced. It requires approximately 5.5 cups of turnip greens to reach your fiber objectives.

Carrots

Steamed carrots will launch more of their beta Carotene; however, whether you like them cooked or raw, you will get all the advantages of 4.68 g of fiber in each cup. It takes about 6 cups of carrots to make it to the fiber intake that is daily.

Cauliflower

Cauliflower is a popular low-carb alternative Vegetable and can be made into chips and pizza crust. It's a great way to add fiber to your diet, but it might not get you to the 28 grams of recommended fiber daily. That might mean eating roughly 8.5 cups of cooked cauliflower, every day.

Fruits

Avocados

Whether in guacamole, on toast, or in salads, avocados are widely enjoyed due to fats and their rich flavor. With 9 grams of fiber each avocado that is medium-size, it might take roughly 3 avocados to attain your daily fiber intake.

Apple

Apples are high in a Sort of soluble fiber called pectin. At 4.4 grams per apple, it takes approximately 7 apples to get your daily fiber. That'll take a while.

Strawberries

Strawberries are also a great source of vitamin C. Slice a Few to get next-level taste and fiber into your salad. You may need to supplement with supplements or other high-fiber foods such as Metamucil--it requires about 6 cups of strawberries to reach the recommended fiber intake, 28 grams.

Banana

Would you consume 9 bananas in a day? One of the most versatile Fruits and a perennial favorite, a banana supplies 3 grams of fiber. Bananas are filling and a fantastic way to add some fiber into a snack or meal.

Raspberries

About two cups of raspberries a day gets you the daily fiber you need. They're a treat that was delicious all by them, baked into your favorite Dessert recipe, or blended at a smoothie.

Nuts & Seeds

Almonds

A serving of almonds contains 3 g of fiber. Attempt

Sprinkling over a few cooked vegetables or entrees to include fiber. It requires approximately 1 cup of almonds to reach on your fiber that is. Milk doesn't, although almond butter contains fiber.

Pecans

Approximately 1 cup of pecans can get one Fiber. Pecans include beta carotene, zinc along with other nutrients that are essential. Top a salad or add a few.

Peanuts

You're not a comfort food Provides a fantastic amount of fiber, particularly once you set it. It requires approximately 1 cup of peanuts to achieve 28 g.

Walnuts

Touted to their walnuts, fats may help should you consume about 2 cups every day you accomplish your fiber targets. Rely on salads and cereals or mix some.

Chia seeds

Chia seeds are well worth adding to your daily diet. High in fiber, they utilized as a crunchy or even a thickener for smoothies. Each tbsp provides 4 grams of fiber.

Legumes

Navy beans

Navy beans are used in soups and baked beans. About 1.5 cups Navy beans can get one to the 28 g per day. Or, make your bean meals a bit "extra" by substituting navy beans to different forms.

Split peas

Approximately 1.5 cups of split peas gets one to the 28 g Of fiber that is. Peas may be utilized as more than just soup. The foundation to get a dish or make a fantastic disperse.

Pinto beans

Creamy pintos will be the bean of choice for producing Refried burritos or beans. Pintos are good as the foundation for burgers. Approximately 2 cups of cooked pinto beans can get you into the daily recommended fiber consumption.

Kidney beans

Beans are a popular in recipes as they maintain their

shape through cooking times and warmth without getting mushy. 1 cup includes 13.1 g of fiber, so consume about two cups of kidney beans to achieve your daily recommended fiber consumption.

Soybeans

With 7.5 g of fiber per cup, they offer amounts of fiber in comparison to other beans. You will want approximately 3.5 cups of cooked soybeans to make it to the daily recommended fiber consumption.

Lentils

Whether you choose brown, yellow, red, or green, lentils are A superb source of fiber. With 15.6 g per cup, you will need about two cups of cooked lentils to make it to the daily recommended fiber consumption. Lentils are excellent as the foundation for burgers or in all types of soups.

Grains

Barley

Does your sugar intake amount to some bowls of soup In winter? Approximately 2 cups of cooked barley daily will get you your daily recommended fiber consumption. Consider adding more plump grain that is high-fiber, of the tender in vegetables, or as a pilaf.

Whole grain pasta

If you are a pasta lover, add up to significant fiber advantages. 1 cup provides 5.46 g of fiber, over twice that of pasta. To achieve your daily recommended fiber intake, then you will need about 5 cups of cooked whole-grain pasta, which might occupy a major part of the suggested quantity of carbohydrates or other nutritional supplements.

Quinoa

Quinoa is packed with 5.18 g of fiber, also with protein per cup, provides 40 percent more fiber than rice. However, it takes approximately 5.5 cups of cooked quinoa to reach the daily recommended fiber consumption. Add quinoa or stir in sugar and cinnamon.

Oats

Great as a cooked cereal, or baked muffins, in cookies, or Granola, oatmeal is high in fiber. It requires about 1 cup of ginger to reach on 28 grams.

Popcorn

Popcorn is a snack that is healthful --but it is going to take 1.5 to you Gallons of popcorn to get the daily fiber consumption. Top it with a scatter of yeast for experimentation or a flavor with spices and your favorite herbs.

Not All Fibers Are Equal -- The Different Kinds Of Fiber And What They Do For Your Entire Body

Fiber is split into two Chief categories, each Wellness and its characteristics advantages. All Kinds of fiber pass through your digestive tract without being digested or absorbed into the blood:

Insoluble

Fiber kind is constructed from big particles. It does not dissolve in water. Fiber can be digested by bacteria during cessation to some degree. If you have large amounts, it may function as a mild laxative by irritating the intestinal lining. Wheat bran is a good illustration of insoluble fiber and many fibrous foods have a part that's insoluble.

Soluble

- Soluble, nonviscous, fermentable: This kind of fiber melts but does not thicken or add bulk to the stool; therefore this fiber isn't successful to be used as a laxative nutritional supplement. It is easily fermented, which is excellent for promoting healthy intestinal flora. But, gas, resulting in flatulence can be produced by fermentation. Examples include dextrin and inulin.

- Soluble Viscous non-fermentable and non-gel-forming: This kind of fiber blends in water. As it isn't fermented and is within feces it helps to boost stool contents. Examples include Methyl-cellulose and Calcium Polycarbophil.

- Soluble, viscous, gel-forming, and fermentable: this kind of fiber grows in water to make a thick gel. This slows the absorption and digestion of glucose and food. It keeps it and protects cholesterol. Therefore this fiber isn't useful as diuretic bacteria consume it, reducing its gel formation. Beta-glucan is and is a good illustration what provides their thick texture to barley and oats. Gum, by the guar bean, is traditionally employed as a commercial food thickener.

- Soluble, viscous, gel-forming, and non-fermentable: This sort of fiber forms a gel, including bulk and water to the stool, but cannot be absorbed by intestinal bacteria, therefore does not cause extra flatulence. Additionally, it helps cholesterol levels and reduces blood glucose *. This fiber is also perfect as a nutritional supplement. It's located from the fiber psyllium, from Metamucil.

High-Fiber Foods

Beans

Legumes and lentils are a Simple way Your daily diet soups, stews, and salads. Some legumes, such as edamame (that can be a steamed soybean), are a fantastic fiber-filled snack. There are g of fiber at a half-cup functioning of edamame. A bonus? All these provide a fantastic source of nourishment. Some bakers have started including bean flours or beans within their goods, which study demonstrates can make standard cakes.

Broccoli

This veggie may get pigeonholed because of the fiber vegetable. Its Character --meaning it is in the Brassica genus of crops together with kale, cabbage, and cauliflower --which makes it rich in nutrients along with fiber. Various studies have demonstrated that broccoli g of fiber can positively encourage the bacteria in the intestine, which might assist your gut to keep healthier and balanced.

Berries

Berries get a Good Deal of attention due to their antioxidants they are filled with fiber. A cup of blueberries may provide you g of fiber, and there is an identical quantity of fiber at a cup of blueberries. Strawberries blackberries and blueberries are also excellent sources of fiber. Obviously, among the advantages of berries is they're naturally low in carbs.

Avocados

Avocados Go Together with everything--salads, toast, Entrees, eggs--and if they are often known for their hefty dose of healthful fats, you will find 10 g of fiber in 1 cup of avocado (so only imagine how much is on your guacamole).

Popcorn

There is also the, and also 1 g in 1 cup of popcorn Snack (when organic rather than coated in butter (such as in the pictures) is a complete grain that may satiate cravings with a bang of fiber. It has been known as the King of Snack Foods.

Whole Grains

News for bread fans: Actual grains, located in 100 percent Whole wheat bread, oats, brown rice, and whole-wheat pasta, have fiber. 1 suggestion to watch out for: as demanded by The Food and Drug Administration, whole grains ought to be the primary ingredient on a food package in order for it to be regarded as a genuine whole grain.

Apples

That old expression that "an apple a day keeps the doctor away" Is not necessarily true, based on a study, however, the fruit may increase your fiber intake. There are approximately 4 g of fiber within an apple, based on its dimensions, however this serving number might help alleviate arteries and reduced cholesterol. And they are a crispy and nice snack.

Dried Fruits

Dried fruits such as prunes, figs, and dates may boost your Fiber consumption drastically and therefore are recommended for those. The sugar called results in more relaxation and will help your intestines. But eating a lot of can cause nausea or cramping, so try a little serving and determine how you feel as soon as you've digested them before noshing on a lot of more.

Potatoes

Sweet red potatoes berries and the Plain old curry are good sources of fiber. The veggie has a reputation for conducting in the audiences --chips and chips, to mention a couple. But slathered in salt and when not fried in oil, potatoes may offer many advantages. The fiber from berries additionally can help to protect the wall.

Nuts

Nuts are a source of healthful and protein Carbohydrates --seeds and sunflower seeds. They will be able to help you arrive at the consumption of fiber recommended by the FDA for girls and recommendation for guys. Steak or dry-roasted nuts have been favored within the prepackaged variety (which is typically cooked in oils which may add extra, unnecessary calories) Nut butters may pack a punch of fiber.

CHAPTER 5
KINDS OF FIBERS

7 Kinds Of Fiber, Explained

You are probably Knowledgeable about the significance of Eating fiber doing this might reduce the chance of developing colon cancer, diabetes, and heart disease. But were you aware that there are many distinct kinds of fiber that each provide their own group of health advantages? (You understand, besides maintaining the amount of two trains on the program.) "Fiber, frequently categorized as 'soluble' (absorbs water through digestion) or' insoluble' (remains unchanged), is really a great deal more complicated," states Connecticut-based registered dietitian Alyssa Lavy, R.D."There are various kinds of fiber under these umbrellas which have different physiological consequences, and in the end, possible health consequences." While water solubility is among the better-known properties of fiber, additional possessions, such as water-holding capability, the capability to bind to

62

additional substances, and the capability of our gut bacteria to ferment fiber efficiently, are significant also. As an instance, some folks can have the ability to tolerate certain kinds of fiber greater than many others, and learning that ones concur with you can make certain you get the best bang for your bran. It is ideal to eat many different foods as a way to eat various kinds of fiber and derive the health benefits. Check out also the foods as well as seven kinds of fiber, ahead.

1. Cellulose

This fiber is a Part of plant cell walls, and vegetables--like broccoli are all sources of cellulose. "Once consumed, cellulose moves through the gastrointestinal tract comparatively undamaged, binding to other food parts you have consumed and helping move things together," states Florida-based registered dietitian Carol Aguirre, R.D... In addition, it keeps the digestive system healthy by helping the development of beneficial gut bacteria (this healthy gut flora is a must in preventing poor bacteria from staging a coup and inducing disease). Additional foods include bran, nuts, and beans.

2. Inulin

Fibers, such as inulin, make you feel fuller for By slowing digestion Further. This also suggests it takes longer for the body to absorb the sugar in the foods which you consume, helping prevent blood glucose spikes (along with also the pesky junk food cravings which could strike because of these). Inulin is not digested or absorbed in the gut --it really sets up shop in the intestines, boosting the development of beneficial flora related to enhancing gastrointestinal (GI) and standard wellness, says Aguirre. (But, it is also a fructan, which is quite fermentable from our gut bacteria, states Lavy, so a few folks may experience GI distress) Inulin is derived from chicory root, also obviously found in veggies and fruits such as peanuts, onions, garlic, and asparagus, in addition to in wheat (such as barley and rye).

3. Pectins

Pectins are Glycemic response of foods by stalling sugar absorption (goodbye, blood glucose spikes!). Our gut bacteria well metabolized them, also such as other fibers, which may help from flushing acids from the body to reduce cholesterol, states Lavy. Pectins are located in large quantities in foods such as strawberries, apples, citrus fruits, carrots, and celery, also in smaller quantities in nuts and legumes.

4. Beta-Glucans

Beta-glucan is Fermentable from our gut bacteria. It is regarded as a prebiotic, supplying"meals" for great gut bacteria, states Edwina Clark, R.D., head of nutrition, and editorial articles in Raised Real. It might be beneficial in increasing satiety and handling blood glucose levels, as a result of properties that delay the speed at which food leaves the stomach and slow transit period inside the intestines, states Lavy. If you would like to rev up your own beta-glucan ingestion, it may be seen in barley, oats, shiitake mushrooms, and reishi mushrooms," says Clark.

5. Psyllium

As a fiber, psyllium helps alleviate constipation by Softening poop pass. Additionally, it creates a handy gel which binds to sugars and also helps to prevent reabsorption of cholesterol from the gastrointestinal tract," says Lauren Harris-Pincus, R.D.N., writer of The Protein-Packed Breakfast Club. (The truth is that it is also a prebiotic that feeds the friendly bacteria in the intestine is merely a bonus.) Since psyllium is the food source -- that the fiber comes from the outer husk of the psyllium plant seeds," states Harris-Pincus--you will only find this kind of fiber for a nutritional supplement or a component added to other foods, including polyunsaturated cereals.

6. Lignin

Lignin is the cell wall structure in crops. Does it perform your research a strong (actually), but a few studies also indicate that insoluble fibers might help to decrease the possibility of developing colon cancer," states Lavy. While the precise mechanism is presently unknown, 1 concept is that it hurries items along from the digestive tract, limiting the total amount of time carcinogens may interact with tissue. Food sources of lignin include whole-grain foods (corn and wheat bran), legumes (beans and legumes), vegetables (green beans, cauliflower, zucchini), fruits (avocado, unripe bananas), along with seeds and nuts (flaxseed).

7. Resistant Starch

"Resistant starch works similarly to soluble, Fermentable fiber, helping feed the friendly bacteria in the intestine," says Aguirre. This implies that it moves to a large intestine, and together with your immune system and microflora, helps safeguard against almost any pathogenic bacteria which tries to mess with your GI tract. In addition, it can assist with weight reduction by taming hunger and blood glucose spikes, heart health by lowering cholesterol, and digestive health by maintaining things every day. Legumes and legumes are great sources of wheat germ, says Aguirre, as are oatmeal flakes and peanuts that have the most amount of starch when they are unripe.

CHAPTER 6
DIFFERENT RENOWNED DIETS
PROGRAMS FOR WEIGHT LOSS

The Top Popular Diets

Fad diets are popular for and a fad Nowadays Losing weight. The aim of these diets is weight loss and health benefits that are many. These diets involve removing foods that contain some nutrients that are vital. Some fad diets cut on the food groups. As an example, foods that are high in protein, low in carbs, or fat-free may be included by fad diets. Some fad diets concentrate on a specific food, like cabbage, grapefruit or beef. Some diets permit you to eliminate specific foods. Diets permit you to eat particular foods, provided that you consume them in conjunction with certain foods. A number of the frequent fad diets that people follow if they're on a weight-reduction plan are ketogenic diet plan, low-fat diet, vegan diet, plant-based diet, Mediterranean diet, Atkins diet, paleo diet and a lot more. Based on nutritionist Monisha, a Delhi-based Nutritionist, "These diets are supposed to provide a jolt to your body making it follow a routine that is different from the typical pattern. So if used it ought to be used for a short duration only!" Delhi based nutritionist Nmami Agarwal said, "Who understood diets also will be trending together with style? And if it's trending, are we following a trend. Well, a response to it stays in the loop gap. Thus, let us try and get the reply to exactly the same and understand if the best two trending diets-"Ketogenic diet" and"Paleo diet plan" are great to be followed or not? Let's get started by talking about the Ketogenic diet plan and know to not be followed and after end up with Paleo diet"

Let's Take a Look in the 10 popular diets:

Raw Food Diet

The raw food diet that is known as raw or raw foodism Veganism focuses on unprocessed and uncooked foods. These foods shouldn't experience processing, not pasteurized be elegant, or treated with pesticides. The diet enables other alternative preparation procedures, including mixing, juicing, dehydrating, soaking and sprouting. So this diet contains a lot and lots of fruits and vegetables. The nutritionist includes, "The raw food diet which contains mainly unprocessed fruits, vegetables, seeds and nuts also has its pros and cons. Processed fruits and vegetables have nutrient material and a higher fiber that has benefits in your health. The diet assists weight loss and limits the consumption of junk and processed foods which are the reason for diabetes and other lifestyle diseases. Cooking makes digestion easier and should raw food it absorbed it may cause gas and bloating. Further, it is helpful to destroy pathogens within the food hence cooking prevents us from getting different foodborne diseases."

Ketogenic Diet

Keto diet, the fad diet is really a low-carb Carbohydrates and moderate in protein diet plan. This diet aids in getting your own body. Ketosis is a condition where your body doesn't have any sugar to burn so that it burns fat rather, and thus assists in rapid weight loss. A number of fats include grape vegetables, poultry yogurt milk plus more. Delhi goes on to state the Keto diet is your FAD Diet that everybody would like to follow. Not intended for everybody, though the diet assists in weight reduction that was enormous. A high-fat diet utilizes ketosis to fuel your body. Ketones are a byproduct of surplus and also metabolism in the human body has results that are detrimental. It can result in fever, flu, and dizziness. Fiber that is vital for the entire body is eliminated by the diet. Fiber keeps you complete and can help prevent cancer of the colon. The diet has to be followed closely with caution. On the flip side, Nmami Agarwal stated"Keto diet may guarantee rapid weight loss but in the price on the health. It may result in hypoglycemia that has low levels of carbohydrates which could result in fatigue, fatigue, and palpations. In addition, it can raise the amount of triglycerides and cholesterol in the human body and such diet may result in fatty liver and constipation in the long term."

Plant-Based Diet

Plant-based diet concentrates on foods as the Name Implies Out of plants. Including not just fruits and vegetables, but also seeds and nuts, oils, whole grains, beans, and legumes.

Mediterranean Diet

The Mediterranean diet besides weight loss is famous Because of its own benefit to cardiovascular health, lowering the chance of cardiovascular disease and enhances the cholesterol level. The diet also lowers the risk of certain cancers in addition to some conditions like Alzheimer's disease and Parkinson's disease.

Atkins Diet

Atkins is among the diets. As a general Thumb rule, it is offered by carbohydrates.

Noom Diet

The Noom program is a weight loss and fitness center program that guides the users of losing weight in addition to the obstacle, through the challenge. The program not only tells you how much you need to exercise and what you ought to avoid, but in addition, it gives the rationale for those practices that are wholesome and information. The diet's aim would be to inculcate wholesome eating habits.

Dubrow Diet

This diet and fasting that means you stick together Eat through the remainder of the moment and throughout a particular period of the day. The diet concentrates exactly what you need to consume and on the length of time you need to.

Carnivore Diet

Meat is included by the carnivore. No carbs vegetables. It may result in nutritional deficiencies as it concentrates on a single food group. A diet devoid of nutrients could be harmful for your health.

Speedy Diet

Fasting is just another plan that trend this year. The theory behind this diet would be to cycle between periods of fasting and eating, where you don't eat any food or remove the calories. Some individuals quickly for a couple hours, though others might quickly for a period per day. The advantages of this fasting could go past weight loss. It assists in metabolism and glucose levels that are steady. The Delhi based nutritionist additionally talks concerning "intermittent fasting where we've got a window of 8 hours to consume and a quick of 24 hours per day. The diet's benefits are in inflammation and that it assists in weight loss. The diet doesn't specify what has to be consumed. That this diet could be helpful for you, if you have. Nevertheless, its negative effects will be shown by excess processed and fast foods, of crap. The most important disadvantage of this is that it may cause excessive acidity that is prone to it"

Paleo Diet

Another diet of this entire year is the Paleo diet. The Paleo diet includes foods that are whole and avoids the foods that are processed. As it avoids the foods that are processed, it is beneficial for shedding those additional kilos. "Paleo is a diet where we normally premise ourselves to consume just what was accessible to Neanderthals from Paleolithic age. Which means removing foods, like sugar and bread and food such as legumes, milk, and grains? Paleo diet gets got the breakdown as fat, very low auto, and large protein. There is no calorie counting with the entire dietary plan and essentially, we consume all of the food items which were available prior to the farming age arrived," explained

Nmami Agarwal. She added, "High protein and low carb diet may result in overeating, lack of energy because of a restriction of carbohydrate. There is also an increased chance of gout and uric acid due to protein addiction from the diet. Still, it may also result in an increased risk of diabetes and Kidney injury"

Popular Diet Plans For Weight Reduction

Balancing food consumption Action is the trick. To Boost energy levels and lead a life that is wholesome, our body demands a proportion of nourishment. There are lots of diet programs - which range that someone may opt for to be able to cut weight. Listed below are our picks of the 6 diets that are hot. Regarded as the Type of vegetarianism, vegan Diet helps in losing weight and thrives on fiber content. This plant-based diet includes health advantages like lower chance of diabetes and heart ailments. This diet is devoid of dairy and meat products. On the reverse side: Sans beef, this diet overlooks important nutrients such as vitamin B12, vitamin D, potassium, iron, calcium, and calcium This protein-based diet includes 100 foods that are split into four stages - assault, cruise, consolidation and stabilization. 2-3 kilos are dropped through protein consumption at the initial phase. In the next phase, the purpose is to attain the weight of pursuing this diet program by eating 28 vegetables. Foods and sugar have been added from the consolidation stage and the purpose is to stop further weight reduction. The final stage is long term and the individual can eat anything he wants to provide specific rules are followed by him. There is a substantial quantity of fat and muscle reduction because the diet demands restrictions. Additionally, it may slow metabolism speed down.

The diet plan's focus is to get rid of carbohydrates Boost and diet intake of fats and proteins. Comparable to this Dukan diet is divided into four stages. From the induction (original) Phase 20 g of carbohydrates is consumed daily for fourteen days. From the rest, the purpose is to healthiest carbs that are wholesome. Being a diet, it may be instrumental in removing belly fat. On the flip side: In rare instances, Health problems can be developed by those like bad breath Dizziness, lethargy, and constipation. Aside from shedding those Additional kilos, this diet may lower the risk of chronic ailments and enhance and Physical wellness. This strategy recommends the ingestion of proteins to get one Part Of the diet along with the remaining veggies and fruits, with a dab of Spread over three foods. And is satisfying Prevents food consumption. On the flip side: Restricts ingestion of healthful Carbohydrates like potatoes, rice, and Bananas. Irregular Fasting The diet a Set of consuming food. It means swallowing calories At length of fasting throughout the remainder and the day. Small Part Of fruits and vegetables are absorbed in periods Dinner at nighttime. With this routine, the calories have been consumed in proportions that were fewer Rather than at the same time. On the flip Facet: This fast-and-feast' strategy may not suit everybody's body cycle and Could be a difficult one. This diet performs wonders Obese or suffers from issues. The Low-carb diet abounds on Foods such as eggs, fish, poultry, legumes, and low carb vegetables. On the flip Facet: Could cause wellness problems such as deficiency, nausea, and desire for sleep.

Best Foods For Dieters

Dieting may be hard Contains foods that you do appreciate. After all, soup that is just how much can a person stand? The fantastic thing is there are hundreds and hundreds of diet foods that are healthful, taste great, and will be able to help you follow your weight loss program. Any supermarket to see the explosion of lower-calorie alternatives.

Here Are only a few Of the top foods for novices:

Calorie-Controlled Snacks. Lots of customers are purchasing the 100-calorie (less or more) bite packs of all chips to cupcakes, but are they the solution for weight reduction? Carolyn O'Neil, RD likes calorie-controlled bundles since they eliminate the opportunity for overeating. "Foods packed in 100-calorie packs do the job and calorie mathematics to you so that you may enjoy snacking on foods which have to be appreciated in restricted quantities," she says. Quaker Mini Delights (90 calories) and Hostess 100-calorie cupcakes are among the addictive choices. However, Lona Sandon, MEd, RD, states that although these snacks may meet a sweet tooth, "most of them won't fill you up for quite long, and can not replace a nutritious bite" Sandon suggests assessing nutrition facts and the ingredient list. "Search for products offering some healthful advantages, like ones which contain greater than 3 g fat, less than 140 mg sodium, 15 g or less sugar, and are produced from whole grain with approximately 2-3 g fiber and approximately 7 g protein," says Sandon, assistant professor in the University of Texas Southwestern Medical Center.

Healthier Fast Food. Fast food restaurants do not need to spell catastrophe for dieters. Attempt Quiznos' Flatbread Sammies without dressing or cheese (less than 250 calories(except that the Italiano) or some little Honey Bourbon Chicken sub (275 calories); Taco Bell's Fresco-style things (less than 180 calories); McDonald's Southwest salad with broiled chicken (290 calories without dressing); or some of Subway's subs with 6 grams of fat or less (230-380 calories).

Low-Fat and Fat-Free Dairy Products. Milk, yogurt (strong, frozen, and tasty), cheese, sour cream, and cream cheese can be found in lower-fat types that provide both wholesome nutrients and fantastic taste. Laughing Cow cheese has wrapped wedge, and Yoplait Fiber One yogurt unites yogurt calories per 4 ounce and cereal to get a fiber increase. Is a substitute for heavy Cream using a fraction? Along with skillet and more lower-fat cream cheese and sour cream may due to their more fatty counterparts, especially. "You can trim calories effortlessly in the event that you utilize low-fat and milder products and whether the item is blended in with other components, nobody will ever see," says Elaine Magee, MPH, RD, and also the "Recipe Doctor" for WebMD plus a WebMD blogger.

Rotisserie Chicken. It is no surprise that nearly every supermarket sells rotisserie chickens. It's possible to function you as can, shred it to use for tacos, pasta dishes, or casseroles, or chop it to get an entree salad. You freeze the meat for a meal debones it and they may get it for supper one night.

Diet-Friendly Desserts. Lower-calorie and portion-controlled candy imply that desserts may be a part of any weight loss diet plan. Dieters who crave ice cream adore Skinny Cow ice cream pops (150 calories), Edy's Slow-Churned ice cream bars (150 calories), also Fudgsicles (100 calories). Fans can appreciate Hershey wafer pubs, vanilla wafers, graham crackers, Fig Newtons, Teddy Grahams, or gingersnaps. On the street, try chewing on a piece of sugarless gum or suck on a piece of hard candy to satisfy your sweet tooth without undermining your diet plan.

Flavored Mustards and Vinegars add sizzle into meals. Try honey, tarragon, ginger, garlic, wasabi, or Dijon mustards, or balsamic, wine, herb, cider, fruit-flavored or, sherry vinegars. Use them.

Light Salad Dressings: Almost half of those salad dressings you will see on your grocer's shelves have been low in fat or calories. Utilize salad spritzers to mist your salads, or try one of light or nonfat salad dressings. Another choice is to produce your dressing, with vinegar than water, in addition to oil.

Cooking Liquids: Dieters have found that wine provides wonderful flavor to stews soups, casseroles, and sauces. Fish, poultry, vegetable, or poultry stocks include a lot of flavor and arrive in types that are fat-free. A key ingredient to add sweetness is orange, apple, or lemon juice concentrate.

Frozen Entrees. This is just another grocery category that has increased as customers search for meals that are easy and quick. Sandon urges the Types including Healthful Option, Lean Cuisine, or Kashi. Read the tag, and search for entries with approximately 300-400 calories, less than 600 mg of sodium, at least 4-5 grams of fiber, and much less than 5 g fat.

Beverages. Great conservative water tops the list of healthful beverages, but if you need something longer, try out these almost calorie-free choices: freshwater waters; powdered packets to combine into bottled water, such as Crystal Light and Propel; green, green, or exotic teas; java; sparkling water; or diet soft drinks. Low-cal options consist of light beer (100 calories/12 oz.); wine spritzers (100 calories/5 ounce); Starbucks' skinny latte or mocha (90 calories/12 ounce); along with the newest V8 juice with fiber (60 calories and 5 g fiber/8 ounce).

Bars. Whether You eat them as meal replacements, or as snacks, pre-workout, these pubs would be the ultimate in convenience. For staying power, start looking for pubs with protein and fiber one pubs.

Dips. Usage These nutritious drops for the own veggies, pretzels, or baked fries for just 5-50 calories per 2 tablespoons: hummus, salsas; succulent black bean dip; mustards; and succulent French onion dip.

Breakfast Cereals. Research indicates that individuals who eat breakfast control their weight better than people who skip the morning meal. Start your day the healthy way using a bowl of whole cereal (high it with low-carb and fruit dairy for additional nourishment). Start looking for cereals with protein and fiber and not too much sugar, such as oatmeal (166 calories, 6 g protein, and 4 g fiber), Kashi Go Lean (140 calories, 10 g fiber, 13 g protein), or Shredded Wheat (155 calories, 5.5 g fiber, 5grams protein).

The Principles For Dieters

Spicy foods are great, but it is difficult to beat the Goodness of whole foods. "Eating more organic, less processed foods is generally a healthier option, but equally may fit into a healthful weight loss diet program," says Sandon.

Here are the four Kinds of food which are the basis of any healthy diet

Lean protein: Lean protein is essential for novices as it enables you to feel fulfilled. Fantastic sources of low carb protein include eggs; skinless poultry, edamame or alternative legumes; nuts; legumes; crab; fish fillets; lean cuts of steak (like filet mignon); and pork tenderloin. Go for cuts, when choosing meat cut all visible fat off, and control your parts. According to the Institute of Medicine's Food and Nutrition Board, you may take% of your calories from protein. So someone within a 1,800-calorie diet may eat around 157 g of protein -- that the equivalent of 1 cup of skim milk, 1 cup cooked black beans, two oz almonds, 1 cup low-fat yogurt, two capsules, 10 oz of fish or meat, and one cup frozen yogurt.

Whole Grains. Whole grains are a fantastic source of fiber, which will help you fill-up. Try out Uncle Ben prepared rice or the pasta combinations. The favored of another dieter is a grain -- crunchy, filling, along with popcorn!

Fruits. They Meet your teeth and are packed with disease-fighting nourishment, however are low in calories. Maintain a stock of fresh, frozen, canned, and dried fruits available, to consume plain or throw into cereal, yogurt, waffles, or batters. Some favorites consist of dried cranberries, berries, and mandarin oranges. Whole fruits are best due to their fiber content, but if you would rather juice, then make sure it is 100% juice and appreciate it in tiny portions.

Veggies. Maintain A source of prewashed mixed greens, shredded carrots, steamed beets, and shredded broccoli slaw available for fast and healthy salads. Roast sweet potatoes for a dish that requires no topping besides a tiny pepper and salt. If vegetables are inclined to become science experiments on your fridge, attempt Birdseye Steamfresh vegetables. Canned vegetables are just another option: simply rinse to decrease sodium. For a bite or the lunchbox, try out the packs of veggie sticks with dip.

CHAPTER 7

7GUT-FRIENDLY

I Am a Gastroenterologist and That Is The Gut-Friendly Meal I Recommend to All My Patients

As Will Bulsiewicz, a gastroenterologist, MD, sees patients with gut health problems that run the gamut, which range from those who find themselves going into the restroom insufficient --the contrary, way too frequently. Regardless of the broad selection of probs, his remedy comes back to a nutrient: fiber. In reality, Dr. Bulsiewicz preaches the value of fiber often to his patients who he is writing a novel on it," Fiber Fueled, so much more people could get schooled on its own function. "We all know our gut microbes certainly thrive when they're fed prebiotic fiber out of actual food," Dr. Bulsiewicz states. "The fiber passes through the gut, unsullied, until it reaches the colon. This sets the microbes that are wholesome. They feast with this yummy meal, then reward you by releasing everything I believe to be the greatest currency of intestine health:

short-chain fatty acids" Dr. Bulsiewicz states that these short-chain fatty acids might help fight leaky gut, fortify the immune system, lower cholesterol, prevent diabetes and protect against colon cancer. (So yeah, they are a fairly major thing.) "They travel as much as your mind to get their health consequences," he states. "And the only real way to get them is when fiber fulfills healthy germs on your colon and gut ensues." With this knowledge that is useful is one thing, but putting it into practice is a whole other. That is why I requested Dr. Bulsiewicz to your supper thought with gut favorable foods that he recommends to each of his patients, so folks can put his intel right into the clinic. His meal full of foods is of the breakfast number Since he is a big believer in starting with gut health in mind.

A Gastroenterologist's Favourite Meal: Oatmeal

Like most other health specialists, "I am a Massive fan of oatmeal," Dr. Bulsiewicz States. "The beauty of this is it's abundant in a prebiotic fiber called beta-glucan that has been demonstrated to enhance the immune system" Also, he enjoys you could add more gut-healthy ingredients with spices and lettuce. While he recommends departing sugar from your bowl (bad germs possess a pleasant sweet tooth) fruits like blueberries (just another G.I. doc's fave gut-healthy meals), strawberries, and peaches have fiber and also include sweetness, whereas nuts boost the fiber material. In terms of spices, he enjoys adding cinnamon, ginger, and garlic for digestion aid. "All three possess anti-inflammatory and advantages in their distinct manner," he states. "Cinnamon helps to keep balanced blood glucose. Ginger has a standing for relieving ailments, and has been proven to help heal the intestine. Turmeric contains a phytochemical called curcumin with some exceptional healing properties, for example shielding the liver and restraining cancer." Additionally, your breakfast is kept by them.

His Second Runner-Up: Smoothies

Another a.m. meal Dr. Bulsiewicz urges: a smoothie." It is a terrific way to sneak a broad mixture of veggies and fruits in your morning," he states. "This is critically important because we understand from Your American Gut Project the single most powerful determinant of a wholesome intestine microbiome is that the diversity of crops on your diet plan. When you boost your plant diversity, then you increase the diversity of your microbiome, also this is a great thing." He typically puts greens, banana, and a couple of frozen berries in his smoothies, however, is based on additional ingredients for taste and fiber functions. "I raise the diversity of crops in my smoothie with the addition of soil flaxseeds, chia seeds, hemp seeds, walnuts, or almonds," Dr. Bulsiewicz states.

Don't Eat

Just urges foods that increase gut health, also, he urges some ones to avoid. "It is just as important to reduce our consumption of foods which encourage inflammatory, unhealthy germs which gas leaky gut," he states. His listing: processed sugars, saturated fat, and artificial sweeteners. Maintain his intel in your mind when constructing smoothie and your oatmeal and your gut will thank you. The key comes down to not just beginning off your day with a fiber-rich meal, but ensuring it is coming from a vast assortment of sources. (Put simply, do not only eat the same old thing daily.) That is why Dr. Bulsiewicz is such a lover of smoothies and oatmeal: both may be customized to taste distinct day daily. Variety is not only the spice of life--it is the trick to good gut health, also.

7 Gut-Friendly Ingredients Also Some Recipes To Use Them Into Enhance Your Gut Health

If You Would like to Shed Weight and feel great, your gut health should be an important part of the way you live. It promotes immunity, keeps your digestive tract routine (yes, which means a normal poo), and is connected with healthy weight reduction. Included in this 28 Day Weight Loss Challenge, we provide recipes and meal plans which can support your weight reduction objectives and, consequently, encourage good gut health.

Here are some easy methods to boost your gut health:

- Cut down on processed foods as they often comprise many ingredients that can upset your stomach

- Cut down sugar (in its many disguises) since it is an inflammatory food

- Make Sure You have Lots of fiber to flush out things and maintain routine

- Consider your use of antibiotics as they kill both good and bad bugs

- Drink plenty of water to flush out your system and also help your body to remove waste

- Permit some germs to get by kissing your pet daily and then to build up your resistance

- From that list, it's easy to see why we do not advocate things such as fatty takeaway, excessive alcohol ingestion, or carbonated cakes at our 28 Day Weight Loss Challenge.

Here Are 7 Of The Most Gut-Friendly Ingredients

Plus some recipes that it is possible to make to assist with your gut health.

1. Greek Yogurt

The bacteria that are is helpful for your gut flora. Blend By attempting these three components with berries to get an antioxidant boosts Yoghurt Berry Ice Blocks.

2. Chia Seeds

High in protein and fiber, they behave as an intestinal irritant To provide a definite out to everything. Consider creating a Berry Chia Pudding before to get an Effortless and quick breakfast. Top with even a dollop of yogurt to get an or blueberries kick.

3. Apple Cider Vinegar

For stimulating the digestion known, this is inserted to your salads with a oil as a dressing table. Also, it functions nicely as a part of recipes such as Sweet and Sour Chicken Meatballs.

4. Gelatine

A supply of protein, also, helps repair the gut lining Look at incorporating some Easy Strawberry Mousse because a dessert choice that is fantastic for your meal plan. Children will love these Homemade Gummy Lollies.

5. Miso

Spicy foods like miso, kefir, and sauerkraut are a fantastic Way to encourage gut health (and they taste great too!). We love adding miso as it provides a great deal of flavor in those Eggs, like for few calories with Miso and Kale.

6. Bananas

All these are an increase, using their fiber Digestion, potassium, and electrolytes to help keep you shooting on all cylinders. For a tasty dessert attempt to get or this 5 Minute Banana Coffee Sundae longer kid-friendly banana recipes.

7. Coffee

Believed to Assist You to digest your food, ginger adds Warmth to stir-fries. Try out this Sesame Ginger Soba Noodle Soup, which also has gut-loving inventory (create your own if you can).

CHAPTER 8
FOODS WHICH ARE HIGH IN
FIBER

7-Day High-Fiber Meal Plan: 1,200 Calories

The strategy to help you lose weight, assist your heart, diabetes risk & make you better. Fiber is a nourishment rock star with some excellent health benefits. Research credits eating more fiber with fat loss, much healthier bowel bacteria, more regularity on your intestine (aka better poops), a wholesome heart, and reduced risk of diabetes. Consequently, if fiber could do this, why are 95 percent of Americans not getting sufficient? Normally, Americans eat 16 g much from the 28 g advocated for Americans. Within this meal program, snacks and your meals for the week are intended for you to make it tasty and easy to get your load of fiber daily. The snacks and meals within this program include lots of fruits, vegetables, whole grains, legumes, seeds, and nuts; in addition to that, but the foods in each class are known to possess the maximum fiber content--believe chickpeas pearshaped, oatmeal, black beans, and chia seeds. Whether you have a couple of ideas from here and there or adhere to this meal program, you will have a far easier time getting the fiber that you want to feel better and stay healthier. Introduce them into your diet, if you are not utilized to eating high-fiber foods and drink water. Eating fiber can cause stomach cramping. We place this strategy with alterations at 1,200 calories each day to bump up this to 2,000 or 1,500 calories, depending upon your needs.

The way to Meal-Prep Your Week of Meals:

- Get Baked Banana-Nut Oatmeal Cups to get for snacks and breakfast during the week.

- Build Brussels Sprouts Salad with Crunchy Chickpeas to get for lunch on Days 2 through 5.

- Make two portions of Apple Cinnamon Chia Pudding to get for breakfast Days 3 & 2.

Day 1

Breakfast (343 calories, 12 g fiber)

- 1 serving Truly Green Smoothie

A.M. Snack (35 Calories, 1 gram fiber)

- 1 clementine

Steak (314 calories, 11 g fiber)

- 1 serving White Bean & Avocado Toast

- 1 small pear

P.M. Snack (105 calories, 2 g fiber)

- 8 dried pine wedges

Dinner (415 calories, 7 grams fiber)

- 1 serving Roasted Chicken & Winter Squash over Mixed Greens

Daily Totals: 1,211 calories, 52 g protein, 162 g carbohydrate, 38 grams fiber, 50 g fat, 1,226 mg sodium

To produce it 1,500 Calories: Insert 1/3 cup dry-roasted unsalted almonds into A.M. snack.

To Produce it 2,000 Calories: Contain all modifications to the 1,500 daily, and boost to 2 servings White Bean & Avocado Toast in lunch, boost to 1/3 cup walnut halves at P.M. bite and include 1/2 an avocado into dinner.

Day 2

Breakfast (233 calories, 10 g fiber)

- 1 serving Apple Cinnamon Chia Pudding

A.M. Snack (176 calories, 3 g fiber)

- 1 serving Baked Banana-Nut Oatmeal Cups

Steak (337 calories, 13 g fiber)

- 1 serving Brussels Sprouts Salad with Crunchy Chickpeas

P.M. Snack (77 calories)

- 1 small apple

Dinner (401 calories, 13 g fiber)

- 1 serving Hearty Chickpea & Spinach Stew

Daily Totals: 1,224 calories, 155-gram protein, 147 g

carbohydrate, 43 grams fiber, 53 g fat, 1,266 mg sodium

To produce it 1,500 Calories: Insert 1 small pear to lunch and two Tbsp. Organic peanut butter into P.M. snack.

To Produce it 2,000 Calories: Contain all alterations for the 1,500 daily, also increase to two servings Baked Banana-Nut Oatmeal Cups at A.M. snack, include 1/2 cup low-fat Greek yogurt into P.M. snack and include 1 serving Guacamole Chopped Salad to supper.

Day 3

Breakfast (233 calories, 10 g fiber)

- 1 serving Apple Cinnamon Chia Pudding

A.M. Snack (35 Calories, 1 gram fiber)

- 1 clementine

Steak (337 calories, 13 g fiber)

- 1 serving Brussels Sprouts Salad with Crunchy Chickpeas

P.M. Snack (154 calories, 3 g fiber)

- 20 dry-roasted, unsalted almonds

Dinner (464 calories, 13 g fiber)

- 1 serving Chicken Fajita Bowls

- 1/4 cup guacamole, for example, Jason Mraz's Guacamole

Daily Totals: 1,223 calories, 67-gram protein, 103 grams carbs, 40 grams fiber, 68 g fat, 1,115 mg sodium

To produce it 1,500 Calories: Insert 1/3 cup dry-roasted unsalted almonds into A.M. snack.

To Produce it 2,000 Calories: Contain all alterations for the 1,500 daily, also add 1 cup low-fat Greek yogurt into breakfast and include two servings Baked Banana-Nut Oatmeal Cups into P.M. snack.

Day 4

Breakfast (259 calories, 3 g fiber)

- 1 serving Baked Banana-Nut Oatmeal Cups

- 1/2 cup low-fat12 plain Greek yogurt

A.M. Snack (131 calories, 7 grams fiber)

- 1 large pear

Steak (337 calories, 13 g fiber)

- 1 serving Brussels Sprouts Salad with Crunchy Chickpeas

P.M. Snack (35 Calories, 1 gram fiber)

- 1 clementine

Dinner (449 calories, 8 grams fiber)

- 1 serving Long-Life Noodles with Beef & Chinese Broccoli

Daily Totals: 1,210 calories, 58 grams protein, 156 g carbohydrate, 32 g fiber, 50 g fiber, 1,253 mg sodium

To produce it 1,500 Calories: Insert 1/3 cup dry-roasted unsalted almonds into P.M. snack.

To Produce it 2,000 Calories: Contain all alterations for the 1,500 daily, also include 1 polyunsaturated English muffin using 1 1/2 Tbsp. Organic peanut butter 1 small apple and include 15 dried walnut halves to A.M. beverage.

Day 5

Breakfast (259 calories, 3 g fiber)

- 1 serving Baked Banana-Nut Oatmeal Cups

- 1/2 cup low-fat plain Greek yogurt

A.M. Snack (77 Calories, 1 gram fiber)

- 10 dry-roasted, unsalted almonds

Steak (337 calories, 13 g fiber)

- 1 serving Brussels Sprouts Salad with Crunchy Chickpeas

P.M. Snack (77 Calories, 4 g fiber)

- 1 small apple

Dinner (465 calories, 10 g fiber)

- 1 serving Slow-Cooker Turkey Chili with Butternut Squash

- 2 cups mixed greens

- 1/4 of an avocado, sliced

- 1 serving Maple Balsamic Vinaigrette with

Shallots

Top blended greens with Chopped avocado and vinaigrette.

Daily Totals: 1,215 calories, 57 g protein, 129 g carbohydrate, 39 grams fiber, 59 g fat, 1,489 mg sodium

To produce it 1,500 Calories: Insert 1 medium apple and add 2 Tbsp. Organic peanut butter into P.M. snack.

To Produce it 2,000 Calories: Contain all alterations for the 1,500 daily, also increase to two servings Banana-Nut Oatmeal Cups and 1 1/4 cups yogurt at breakfast and boost to 1/3 cup dry-roasted unsalted almonds into A.M. snack.

Meal-Prep Tip: Book 2 servings Slow-Cooker Turkey Chili with Butternut Squash to get for lunch on Days 7 & 6.

Day 6

Breakfast (343 calories, 12 g fiber)

- 1 serving Truly Green Smoothie

A.M. Snack (16 Calories, 1 gram fiber)

- 1 cup sliced lemon

- Pinch of pepper & salt

Steak (311 calories, 14 g fiber)

- 1 serving Slow-Cooker Turkey Chili with Butternut Squash

- 1 clementine

P.M. Snack (37 calories, 2 g fiber)

- 1 medium bell pepper, sliced

Dinner (505 calories, 11 g fiber)

- 1 serving Butternut Squash Alfredo with Chicken & Spinach

Daily Totals: 1,212 calories, 71-gram protein, 148 g carbohydrate, 40 grams fiber, 42 g fat, 1,718 mg sodium

To Produce it 1,500 Calories: Insert 1 whole-wheat English muffin using 1 1/2 Tbsp. Peanut butter.

To Produce it 2,000 Calories: Contain all alterations for the 1,500 daily, and include 1/4 hummus and 1/3 cup dry-roasted unsalted almonds to A.M. bite and include 1/4 cup guacamole into P.M. snack.

Meal-Prep Tip: Marinate the pork for Roasted Pork Tenderloin with Vegetables & Quinoa therefore it is ready for supper tomorrow.

Day 7

Breakfast (259 calories, 3 g fiber)

- 1 serving Baked Banana-Nut Oatmeal Cups

- 1/2 cup low-fat plain Greek yogurt

A.M. Snack (37 calories, 2 g fiber)

- 1 clementine

Steak (311 calories, 14 g fiber)

- 1 serving Slow-Cooker Turkey Chili with Butternut Squash

- 1 clementine

P.M. Snack (101 Calories, 6 grams fiber)

- 1 medium pear

Dinner (490 calories, 8 grams fiber)

- 1 serving Italian Roasted Pork Tenderloin with Vegetables & Quinoa

Daily Totals: 1,198 calories, 72-gram protein, 153 g carbohydrate, 33 grams fiber, 37 g fiber, 1,600 mg sodium

To produce it 1,500 Calories: Insert 1/3 cup dry-roasted unsalted almonds into P.M. snack.

To Produce it 2,000 Calories: Contain all alterations for the 1,500 daily, also increase to two servings Baked Banana-Nut Oatmeal Cups and boost into 1 cup yogurt at breakfast and include 1 whole-wheat English muffin with 1 1/2 Tbsp. Organic peanut butter into A.M. snack.

High-Fiber Meals To Add To Your Diet (And Fiber Is So Great In The First Place)

You know that fiber is also an important component of a healthy diet. But let us be honest: Do you understand what fiber is? Let us ask a dietitian. "Fiber is your nondigestible portion of plant foods which can be found in whole fruit and vegetables, seeds, nuts, whole grains and legumes such as greens, lentils and peas," says registered dietitian Brynn McDowell. Fiber is broken down into 2 classes: soluble fiber, that dissolves in water and maybe divided up from the bacteria in our intestine, and fiber, which adds mass to our feces and doesn't dissolve, McDowell describes. Both are important to our everyday diet since fiber helps regulate blood sugar, lower cholesterol, and feed the good bacteria in our intestine, decrease the chance of cardiovascular disease, prevent constipation and also allow you to feel (and remain) full after ingestion. Nutrition guidelines state that women below 50 years old ought to consume 25 grams of fiber every day, while girls over 50's age should target for 21 grams daily. And getting sufficient fiber is critical. "Low dietary fiber consumption may result in poor digestive health, which means increased risk for constipation, diverticular disease, and migraines," McDowell says. "Cholesterol levels in the blood may also grow, which may result in an increased risk for both cardiovascular disease and stroke. A diet low in fiber means that a diet low in fruits and vegetables, whole grains, beans, and legumes. Besides being low in fiber, this may also indicate a diet lacking in a variety of nutrients, minerals, and vitamins." Yikes. The excellent

106

news is that incorporating foods is straightforward. 1 cup of berry contains eight grams of fiber, a cup of whole-wheat java has six grams plus half a cup of legumes contains 7.5 grams. Additionally does not need to be complex. "I advise taking a look at your present foods and seeing how you can incorporate more fiber to what you're eating," McDowell informs us. "For instance, selecting 100 percent whole-wheat bread on white bread increases the fiber material. Adding a few fresh berries and chopped almonds into yogurt, placing a spoonful of chia seeds or flaxseed in your morning smoothie, or adding beans to soups or chili are simple actions you may take from the kitchen to include more fiber into your foods." Do it when increasing fiber in your diet and make sure you increase your water consumption.

Salmon Bowl With Farro, Black Beans And Tahini (27g Fiber)

Every element of the recipe contains fiber in the two Tablespoons of tahini from the dressing have nearly 3 grams of fiber, along with the avocado and lettuce adds yet another boost.

Veggie Nicoise Salad With Red Curry Green Beans (7g Fiber)

Salads are high in fiber, but this riff on the Salad that is Classic adds additional with beans.

Harissa Chickpea Stew With Eggplant And Millet (35g Fiber)

Millet is a fiber enthusiast that is comparatively unsung. This entire grain Packs in 2 grams per 100 g serving, and it is as yummy we promise. Let those hot stew flavors soak up and you will be hooked.

Chickpea And Vegetable Coconut Curry (32g Fiber)

Chickpeas are packed with fiber, and also the more veggies you Add to the curry, the length of that stuff that is fantastic you will eat.

Creamy Vegan Lentil And Roasted Vegetable Bake (11g Fiber)

Veganizing fiber in which is added by this dish using cashew cream Dairy would be, along with an excess dash is added by the nuts on top.

Lemon Tahini Salad With Lentils, Beets And Carrots (19g Fiber)

The real key to turning any salad? Add lentils. They are chock full of fiber (which fills up you (as you currently know).

The Supreme Quinoa Avocado Bowl (13g Fiber)

By now, you are likely well acquainted with all our buddy quinoa. It is not a grain, it is a seed, so it's lots of protein while packing in an impressive quantity of fiber.

Soba Noodles With Peanut Sauce (8g Fibers)

Made from buckwheat soba noodles are a high-fiber Alternative to bread noodles. Peanuts have a nice level, as do legumes.

Buckwheat Gnocchi With Cabbage, Potatoes And Fontina (6g Fiber)

If you are eager to get a job Gnocchi, created with ricotta cheese, ought to be it. Potatoes are also a source of fiber, together with roughly 5 g in one potato. Add cabbage and more greens to up the fiber.

Avocado, Radish And Walnuts With Carrot-Miso Dressing (13g Fibers)

This salad seems like it came from a restaurant Kitchen, but it simple to create. Grab your great knives, slit, and build.

Portobello Mushrooms Stuffed With Barley Risotto (10g Fiber)

Mushrooms are reduced in Along with becoming fiber powerhouses Carbohydrates, fat, and carbohydrates. Stuff that portobello with more fiber in the kind of creamy grains. 1 bite and you will forget you aimed to get healthful.

Sweet Potato And Black Bean Nachos With Green Chili Salsa (10g Fiber)

Swapping chips out for crispy potatoes is a and Yummy move to include fiber. The tomatillo salsa additionally and bean topping add the dish and fiber.

Spicy Chili Crisp White Bean And Barley Stew With Kale And Eggs (14g Fiber)

Chili amps up the spiciness of the vegetarian stew That

is packed with ingredients. (Insert a side of edamame and brown rice to get much more.)

Vegetarian Stuffed Peppers (7g Fiber)

The meals arrive in bowls. These stuffed peppers Are super simple to create, and should you sub the rice for brown rice or another whole grain (cook it a bit first), then you are going to add much more.

CHAPTER 9
HIGH-FIBER RECIPES FOR
BREAKFAST

High Fiber Breakfasts To Help Meet Your Recommend Intake

If you have ever said "I am not a breakfast person," you Could be missing out. Breakfast is a chance to begin on the nutrient that is strong footing. If you are attempting to get more fiber in your diet breakfast is a fantastic means to do that. Fiber is found in fruits, vegetables, grains, and seeds, according to the most recent version of the USDA Dietary Guidelines. And why would you want this carbohydrate that is magical? Well, studies have revealed that fiber lessens the risk of cardiovascular disease and may encourage gut health. Most adults must be getting somewhere between 22 and 34 g of fiber every day, however, research shows many people are falling short. To assist you to meet the daily recommended amount of fiber, and then we have collected up 19 fast recipes which package in 5 to 50 g per serving.

High Fiber Breakfast Smoothies

Raw Banana Cacao Breakfast Smoothie

Cacao powder is your source of fiber within this luscious smoothie. 1 tablespoon has 2 grams of fiber, and this recipe also calls for 2 tbsp. You can do the math. Whirl it up along with other yummy sources of fiber, such as banana, dates, almond milk, and almond butter and you would swear it is not healthy.

This Banana Cacao Breakfast Smoothie is packed with super and taste foods to get a hearty and tasty breakfast.

Ingredients

- 1 frozen banana, sliced

- Two Medjool dates, pitted

- 2 tablespoons raw almond butter

- 2 tablespoons raw cacao powder

- 1 tablespoon chia seeds

- 1 cup uncooked almond milk

Instructions

- Toss all ingredients in a blender and blend on high until smooth.

Pb&J Smoothie

Frozen strawberries (a sub for keratin) supply about 5 g Butter, and of fiber per cup adds yet another 3 g. Like an entire banana and 2 heavy spoonfuls of peanut butter weren't sufficient, this recipe includes some ginger and chia seeds also. The outcome is a using a high fiber count.

Ingredients

- 1 ripe banana, chopped or whole

- 1 cup frozen berries

- 1/4 cup fermented rolled oats (not quick-cooking!))

- 2 tbsp peanut or almond butter

- 1 tbsp chia seeds

- 1/2 cup unsweetened almond milk

- 1 tsp honey or agave (discretionary)

Instructions

- Add all of the ingredients and mix until smooth!

Triple-Berry Chia Detox Smoothie

Three Types of package this smoothie with Fiber. It is going to keep in the refrigerator for 3 to 4 times, which makes it effortless to begin the day with great moral fiber (ha -- determine exactly what we did there?). Here is the lowdown on fiber each cup: Raspberries consume 16 g, blackberries have approximately 8 g, and berries have approximately 5 g. Insert chia seeds and two bananas and you are getting a wholesome dose of fiber into an irresistible beverage.

Description

Complete Time: 15 minutes

Prep: 15 minutes

Cook: 0 minutes

Yield: 6 servings

Amount: Easy

Ingredients

- 1/4 cup chia seeds

- 2 cups water

- 2 cups organic frozen berries, thawed

- 2 cups organic frozen blackberries, thawed

- 1 1/3 cups organic frozen raspberries, thawed

- 2 large bananas, peeled and cut into thirds

- 1/4 cup agave (discretionary)

Instructions

- Insert water and the chia seeds and stir fry until all seeds are soaked. Set the bowl in the fridge.

- Meanwhile, add the berries, blackberries, raspberries, bananas, and agave (discretionary) into a food processor or blender. Pulse until ingredients are pureed.

- Eliminate in the refrigerator. The chia seeds ought to have absorbed the majority of the water. Insert the chia mix until well blended and pulse. Drink immediately.

- **Storage:** Smoothie will maintain up for 3-4 days when stored in the fridge in an airtight container. Part individual portions of this smoothie into freeze and containers; thaw in the refrigerator.

Straight Forward Pumpkin Spice Smoothie

With this particular, Begin Rather than a pumpkin spice latte fiber-rich smoothie. As a result of this material available year-round, there is no need. A cup of pumpkin puree contains 7 grams of fiber. When pumpkin joins forces with spinach and chia 14, Along with the fiber count develops. I adore this smoothie for autumn days. Pumpkin is a high Perfect for removal and digestion.

INGREDIENTS

- 1 1/2 cups unsweetened almond milk or plain water

- 7 ounce fresh, roasted pumpkin puree (or 1/2 15 ounce can)

- 1/2 cup lettuce

- 1 tsp vanilla extract

- 1/2 teaspoon no sugar spice

- 1 tablespoon chia seeds

- Discretionary: pumpkin seeds

INSTRUCTIONS

- Blend all ingredients. Sprinkle with pumpkin seeds. Enjoy!

High Fiber Breakfast Pubs

Quinoa Breakfast Pubs

Whip these on a Sunday morning and you'll have Breakfasts for the week. Half cups of quinoa include the pan and 18 grams of fiber and 36 g of protein together. Um... yes, please. Chia seeds nuts and peanut butter bring fiber into those yummy treats.

INGREDIENTS

- 1 c whole wheat germ (or chickpea flour to Generate GF)

- 1.5 c cooked quinoa

- 2 coats

- 1/2 c nuts, chopped

- 1 teaspoon cinnamon

- 1 teaspoon baking soda

- 2 Tbsp chia seeds

- 2/3 c peanut butter

- 1/2 call honey

- 2 eggs

- 2/3 c applesauce (or mashed banana)

- 1tsp vanilla

- 1/3 c craisins

- 1/3 c chocolate chips (optional)

INSTRUCTIONS

- Combine quinoa, applesauce, vanilla, eggs, peanut butter, and honey in a bowl and combine well.

- Add the remaining ingredients and stir until blended.

- Spoon into a greased 9×13 pan and bake at 375 or till golden brown.

- Let cool and cut into bars.

- Store in the fridge.

Apple Flax Breakfast Squares

Without flour in sight, these sweetened, Treats that are spice-infused rely upon 3 cups of ground flaxseeds. And do these seeds deliver! 1 cup includes 46 grams of fiber. Better still, this recipe makes 12 servings, which means you are all set for the week (and next week, even should you freeze a few).

Ingredients

- 3 cups (336g) ground flaxseed (also called flaxseed meal)

- 2 tsp baking powder

- 2 tsp cinnamon

- 1/2 tsp nutmeg

- 1/2 tsp salt

- 1/2 cup unsweetened apple sauce

- 1/2 cups maple syrup

- 4 eggs

- 2 tsp vanilla extract

- 1/4 (48g) cup + 1 tsp melted coconut oil

- 1 apple, peeled, cored, and sliced

- 1/2 cup walnuts, walnuts, or pecans chopped.

Instructions

- Preheat oven to 350 degrees. Grease a 9 x 13 (quarter sheet) pan with 1 teaspoon of the melted coconut oil.

- Blend salt powder, cinnamon, nutmeg, and ground flaxseed.

- Insert maple syrup, the apple sauce, eggs, and vanilla extract and blend well.

- Stir in the coconut oil then fold in nuts and the apple.

- Spread mixture evenly in the pan. Bake for thirty minutes at the bottom rack of the oven.

- Let cool then cut to squares/rectangles.

High Fiber Breakfast At A Bowl

Chia Seed Skillet

This breakfast gets its remaining power. Require 2 minutes to blend and wake up to a meal you'll be fueled by that and them together. One contains 1/8 cup. Fruit will increase the fiber count. A cup of banana can include nearly two g of fiber.

Ingredients

- 1/4 cup chia seeds

- 1.5 - 2 cups milk from your selection (soy, almond, coconut, hemp, etc..)

- 2 tbsp pure maple syrup

- 1 tsp vanilla

Instructions

- Mix all ingredients in a bowl, whisk to reduce clumping. Or mix all ingredients with a blender.

- Note: For a pudding that is milder, reduce the quantity of milk utilized.

- Shop in an air-tight container and refrigerate.

- Serve with toppings of your choice! Mangos, bananas, berries, kiwi, walnuts, almonds, cinnamon, maple syrup, pineapple, etc..

Easy And Quick Sweet Brown Rice Skillet

There is no reason that this grain that is fiber-riffic cannot take Centre point on your breakfast. Half a cup of brown rice contains 1.5 grams of fiber. That the fiber count is upped by A apple.

INGREDIENTS

- 1/2 cup unsweetened vanilla almond milk

- 1 Tbsp. pure maple syrup

- 1 Tbsp. almond butter

- Two Medjool dates, sliced

- 1 medium apple, peeled, cored, and diced

- 2 cups cooked brown rice

- 1/2 tsp. cinnamon

INSTRUCTIONS

- In a saucepan combine dates, maple syrup butter, milk, and apple. Bring to a boil, stirring to avoid burning, and make sure that everything is well blended. Reduce heat to low and cook for approximately 5 minutes until apple and dates have softened.

- Add cooked cinnamon and rice, stirring until the ingredients are combined. Keep on cooking for approximately 5 minutes, until rice is soft and warm. Drink immediately.

Delicious Mocha Oatmeal

Why don't you set on your oatmeal? It is a lot Fitter than even a bowl or the usual mochaccino. And it takes only 7 minutes to pull on at this breakfast together. The oats supply 6 g of fiber, so the walnuts have two grams of fiber, and also 3 g are added by a banana. This adds up to greater than 10 g of fiber.

Ingredients

- 1 banana

- 3/4 cup porridge oats

- 1 teaspoon instant coffee

- 1/4 teaspoon salt

- 1 teaspoon honey

- 1/2 tsp cacao powder

- 1 cup water

- 1/4 cup walnuts

- 1 cup milk, additional when functioning (can be soy, almond, rice, anything you like -- only keep it fermented if desired)

Instructions

- Prove your strength - peel squash your banana.

- Set, coffee powder, cacao powder, salt, sausage, and banana.

- Insert the cup of water.

- Let it simmer till it takes on a feel.

- Chuck to a bowl, and then add honey and the milk.

- Or plan and prepare yourself oats. Verify the notes.

Blueberry Fiber Starter

We would not dream of taking away your cereal, but here is a recipe that is great to present your Cheerios a run for their money. Three types of seeds electricity that this breakfast. Sunflower (2 g of fiber), chia, hemp (less than a gram), and flax (2 g). Now that is a bowl we could get on board.

INGREDIENTS

- 1/2 cup tomatoes or sliced apple

- 2 tablespoon hemp seeds

- 2 tablespoon chia seeds

- 2 tablespoon sunflower seeds

- 1 tbsp ground flax seeds

- 2 cups vanilla milk

INSTRUCTIONS

- Combine the first five ingredients in a bowl. Pour almond milk. Allow the bowl to sit for 2-3 minutes before serving to enable the liquid to be absorbed by the chia seeds and enlarge.

Vanilla And Fig Overnight Oats

New dates sweeten this bowl of oatmeal and figs -- and one cup of oats has 8 grams of fiber. Chia seeds' sprinkling and the bowl add about a gram all fiber and protein together.

Serves 2

- 2 cups rolled oats

- 2 cups vanilla milk, unsweetened

- 1 vanilla bean pod

- 1 Tablespoon chia seeds

- 3 dates, pits removed

- 4 new figs

METHOD:

- In a bowl or a jar put input aside and rolled oats and chia seeds.

- Pod lengthwise split. Gently scrape out the small seeds. Add to blender dates the milk, and figs and mix until mixture is incorporated.

132

- Pour vanilla milk & on the fig and stir to blend. Cover and refrigerate overnight.

- At the morning oats using nuts, figs, and a spoonful of honey if desired. Enjoy!

Savory Oatmeal With Figs, Pine Nuts, And Feta Cheese

Do not rule out should you prefer salty to sweet in the morning oatmeal. In this recipe, our treasured breakfast grain that is fiber-rich begins with 8 g of fiber per cup. The Mediterranean flavors of figs, feta, and nuts are good. Bookmark this one for the following "breakfast for dinner" nighttime.

Ingredients:

- 2 cups water

- 1 cup organic thick rolled oats

- 6 dried palmyra figs, diced

- 2 tbsp pine nuts, raw or lightly toasted in a skillet

- 1/4 cup crumbled feta cheese, or more to taste

- Extra virgin olive oil- to flavor

- Fresh ground pepper (I used a combination of pink and black peppercorns whom I ground coarsely in a mortar and pestle)- to flavor

Instructions:

- Water on high heat in a medium saucepan and figs. Bring to a boil, and then reduce heat and cook, stirring occasionally, till the water is merely about consumed (approximately 5 minutes). Allow to cool slightly

- Spoon the oatmeal into serving bowls and top with feta cheese and the pine nuts. Drizzle in some olive oil and top with the black pepper.

High Fiber Breakfast Chief Dishes

Chickpea Flour Breakfast Pizza

This breakfast is kept by A flour Gluten-free and high in fiber. A serving of garbanzo bread contains 5 g of fiber. Top with salsa, avocado, and lettuce and you are taking a Look Powerhouse of nutrients which you deserve to create for yourself.

INGREDIENTS

For the crust:

- 1/3 cup garbanzo bean flour

- 1/3 cup water

- 1/4 tsp garlic powder

- 1/8 teaspoon salt

- Pepper, to taste

For the toppings:

- 2 eggs, beaten

- 3--4 tablespoons salsa

- 1/4 of an avocado, cubed

- Sliced green onions, for serving

INSTRUCTIONS

- Heat a pan sprayed with cooking spray over medium heat. In a small bowl, stir together garbanzo bean flour, water, garlic powder, salt, and pepper.

- Pour batter into the pan and cook for approximately 6 minutes. Flip and cook for another four minutes (the crust must be quite simple to reverse --or even, allow it to cook a few minutes more).

- Remove from pan. Spray on the pan and add eggs. Scramble until place.

- Spread salsa over crust. Add scrambled cubed avocado, eggs, and green onions. Season with pepper and salt and serve!

Make-Ahead Breakfast Quesadilla With Cheese, Lettuce, Along With White Beans

We have never met with we did not enjoy, but let us face although an It, many restaurant variations do not just scream "healthy" This recipe makes eight quesadillas full of legumes, eggs, and eggs. Along with ooey-gooey cheese -- we could not forget that. Tortillas are the chief source of fiber. Beans are a wonderful source with approximately 13 g per cup. And though every tortilla is dispersed with less than two oz, we will take it.

Ingredients

- 10 large eggs

- 1 tbsp milk

- 1/2 tsp kosher salt

- 1/2 tsp garlic powder

- 1/2 tsp black pepper

- 1/2 tablespoon peppermint oil

- 5 cups lightly packed fresh spinach - about torn or sliced (about 4 oz)

138

- 1 May reduced-sodium white beans - (15 oz), like cannellini, Great Northern, or white kidney, rinsed and drained (I normally use cannellini)

- 1 1/2 cups freshly grated cheese - like cheddar, Swiss, mozzarella, or another comparable melty cheese; I adore sharp white cheddar (approximately 5 oz)

- 8 whole-wheat tortillas - moderate taco dimensions, about 7 inches

Instructions

- In a large bowl whisk together the eggs, salt, milk, garlic powder, and pepper. Put aside.

- Add the olive oil into a large nonstick skillet over moderate heat until it's warm and shimmers. Swirl to coat the pan, then add the spinach and cook, stirring frequently, until it starts to wilt, about 1 minute. Add the beans; decrease the heat to medium-low pour in the eggs. Using a rubber spatula, cook the eggs slow and low, with the spatula to maneuver them around the pan frequently. Keep on cooking until the eggs are set,

139

about 5 minutes, and scrambled. Taste and season with additional salt or pepper as desired. Remove from heat. (If freezing the quesadillas, allow the filling cool entirely.)

- To build the quesadillas: Sprinkle a tortilla using one-eighth of the shredded cheese, leaving a small border around the border. Spoon one-eighth of this egg mixture at the top, and then fold the tortilla in half. Repeat with the remaining tortillas.

- **To cook quickly:** Gently wipe out the skillet. Increase the heat to moderate and gently coat the skillet with nonstick spray (or brush with a little bit of further olive oil). Cook the constructed quesadillas on either side till golden and the cheese is melted, about 5 to 6 minutes total. Cut into wedges and serve hot.

- To freeze allow the egg filling cool to room temperature. Once chilled, form the quesadillas as mentioned above, then wrap every built quesadilla separately in plastic wrap. Organize the quesadillas in one layer on a baking sheet or similar level surface which will fit on your freezer. Place the sheet in the freezer before the quesadillas are business, then move them into a freezer bag or airtight container. Freeze for up to 2 weeks. To cook from frozen, remove the plastic wrapping and then warm the quesadilla from the microwave for 2-3 minutes until heated through. As an alternative, you can allow them to thaw overnight in the fridge and cook in a skillet directed above.

Notes

Watch recipe instructions for notes freezing the quesadillas. You may even keep the egg filling individually in the fridge for up to 3 times, and then build the quesadillas before cooking. I don't suggest storing assembled quesadillas from the fridge, as the tortillas may get mushy.

Coconut Banana Sandwiches

You had us pancakes because What Type of listing would this be with them? Coconut flour is your astonishing fiber source inside this banana pancake for you -- only 1/4 cup contains 10 g of fiber.

Ingredients

- 4 egg whites

- 1/2 big ripe banana, carrot

- 1/3 cup unsweetened almond milk

- 1/4 tsp almond extract (optional)

- 1/4 cup coconut milk

Instructions

- Preheat a skillet or griddle to medium heat and coat with cooking spray. *

- Whisk egg whites till frothy.

- Add remaining ingredients and stir well.

- Spoon batter onto skillet, forming 4 polyunsaturated pancakes, and let to

- Cook 5-6 minutes each side before turning.

- Coating and plate with half banana, toasted a spoonful of butter, and coconut.

Rustic Sweet Curry Breakfast Decoration

Next time you bake sweet potatoes an up one-two -- which means this recipe can rustle up. This hash comes together with berries, spinach and potato topped with an egg that will induce you to lunch, in moments. We are about getting in certain love first thing in the afternoon. 1 sweet potato has about 3 g of fiber. To up the material, sprinkle with a tablespoon of ground flaxseeds or sunflower seeds.

INGREDIENTS

- 1 small sweet potato

- 1/4 cup cereal

- 1/4 cup lettuce, frozen or fresh

- 1/4 cup tomato

- 1 egg

- Turmeric powder

- Pepper

- Cooking spray

*amounts could easily Be corrected for taste, and Number of individuals.

INSTRUCTIONS

- Utilize a potato you cooked or prepare. To prepare you - check for softness, poke a fork, then loosely wrap in a paper towel clean, reverse it and return it. Do not over-cook it or it'll get rough. Let it cool and then dice to 1/4 inch bits.

- Spray a skillet in which you have a lid and place to begin to brown them over medium or medium-high.

- While that's cooking dice a few onion, then cut on a few curry, and then extract your lettuce.

- Transfer your potatoes and be certain that they're browning. Add the onion. As soon as they begin to brown add your spinach. Permit it wilt if new, if frozen or defrost.

- Before you're ready to set your egg add the tomato, a dash of garlic and pepper powder stir the mix.

- Push on everything. Carefully and attentively

crack your egg(s) along with the hash. Set immediately. Let it cook 1- 2 minutes with yet another 3-5 with it and warmth off. The egg should be cooked by the warmth within the pan. Test if the egg isn't cooked to your taste, it might require extra time or using the lid.

Avocado Toast With Spiced Skillet Chickpeas

Avocado toast is on menus nowadays, however this staple Variant is a WOW. Smoky maple chickpeas include a pinch, also fiber, and protein. A can of chickpeas contains 16 grams of fiber.

Bonus: You will have for snacking chickpeas.

INGREDIENTS

Chickpeas:

- 16oz may or box of chickpeas, drained/rinsed

- 1 teaspoon garlic

- 1 teaspoon smoked paprika

- 1 1/2 Tbsp lemon juice

- 1-2 tsp maple syrup, tier B

For the pan: 1 teaspoon extra virgin olive oil (use longer to get longer succulent chickpeas)

- 2 large chopped sourdough bread, toasted (utilize any bread)

- 1 avocado, sliced for mashing

- 2 tsp chopped parsley or cilantro

- Lemon wedges on the side

- Drizzle of EVOO on the top to function

INSTRUCTIONS

- Warm a skillet over high heat and put in the extra virgin olive oil. Add the drained chickpeas when oil is hot. Shake the pan. Half the spices on top of the chickpeas. Let them sit sizzling in the pan for 1-2 minutes; shake the pan the chickpeas must be coated with the yellowish and crimson spices. Add the lemon juice and maple syrup and then shake around the pan. Add in another half of these spices and then shake the chickpeas to disperse. Keep shaking for the minutes since you let the chickpeas to brown and cook, absorbing the tastes. If the chickpeas have toasted round the borders a little and are well in color -- they are finished. Sprinkle the sea salt on top. Put aside.

- Toast the bread and with a fork, then smash on the avocado. Sprinkle the chickpeas add the parsley or cilantro garnish and drizzle EVOO on top to function. Serve with lemon wedges as you consume, and squeeze lemon on top. Slice and serve!

Peanut Butter Flaxseed Pancakes

All these pancakes that are no-dairy utilize flaxseeds' gelling Ability to substitute an egg. Oat flour provides 3 g of fiber to every pancake, and wheat germ adds another 2 g. everything adds up in a great way.

Ingredients

- 1 batch ginseng egg (1 Tbsp (7 grams) flaxseed meal + 2 1/2 Tbsp (37 ml) water since initial recipe consists of // or sub poultry egg)

- 1 Tbsp Earth Balance (melted // or alternative non-dairy butter)

- 1/2 cup unsweetened vanilla almond milk

- 1 Tbsp agave nectar or maple syrup (or honey to get non-vegan)

- 1 teaspoon baking powder

- 1/2 tsp baking soda

- 1 Tbsp organic unsalted peanut butter (creamy or crunchy // and additional for topping)

- 1 pinch salt

- 1/2 teaspoon pure vanilla extract

- 1/2 cup oat flour

- 1/4 cup whole-wheat pastry flour

Instructions

- Preheat electric griddle to medium heat (roughly 350 degrees F / 176 C), or even a large skillet on the stovetop. You want the surface to become hot but not yelling hot -- when it leaves contact oil should not smoke.

- To a large bowl include water and coriander and let sit for 2 or a moment. Add melted Earth Balance, agave nectar, peanut butter, baking soda, baking powder, salt, vanilla extract, and whisk to blend. Add milk and whisk until well blended.

- Next, add wheat pastry and oat flour and stir until blended. Let batter rest for 5 minutes.

- Grease your griddle and pour cup dimensions of the batter. There should be 6 pancakes (as the first recipe is composed). Flip when bubbles appear in the edges and the center turns tender, being careful not to burn.

- Cook for 1-2 minutes longer on the other hand and top with Earth Balance or even more peanut butter and a drizzle of maple syrup, or anything else you please.

- Will reheat well from the microwave.

*Nutrition Info is a rough estimate.

High-Fiber Lunch Recipes

Most of us know that the three p.m. slump far also. Lunch was a fast Piece of pizza since we were too busy to prep a salad. We're hungry and we will eat anything. Hello, cupcakes in the kitchen. What that pizza was lost was (other) favorite f-word: fiber. You know that substance found in fruits and vegetables that keeps you regular and lessens the chance of disease. If the term "fiber-filled" conjures up pictures of dull old cereal, then fear not. You are excited to begin bringing your lunch to work once you understand food is this freakin' fantastic.

High Fiber Lunch Salads

Honey Mustard Salmon With Shaved Brussels Sprout Salad

This recipe is a fun way to change your packaged Salad regular. The brussels sprouts are a filling, higher fiber choice to lettuce, whereas the grilled salmon has to be served room temp, so it is perfect at the office.

INGREDIENTS

- 4 Salmon Filets

- 2 tbsp Honey

- 2 tbsp Dijon Mustard

- Juice from little lemon

- Salt and pepper to taste

Salad:

- 16 oz of Brussel Sprouts, shaved

- 1 little Fuji Apple, chopped thin.

- 2 tbsp rice wine vinegar

- 1 tsp honey

PREPARATION

- Preheat broiler. Combine Dijon mustard, honey, and lemon juice to get salmon filets. Coat all filets and place them in the broiler for approximately 5 minutes or till brown and cooked.

- In a different bowl mix rice vinegar and honey. Toss together Brussel sprouts and apples.

- Permit salmon to cool before putting along with your sprout salad!

154

5-Minute Lentil Tomato Salad

Do not you hate foods that require longer preparation than they Do to consume? This is not among these. It takes all of 5 minutes to throw fried broccoli, chubby cherry tomatoes, and chives in a bowl. Keep it simple with vinegar and salt, or require an additional 30 minutes to throw in garlic and some chopped ginger for flavor.

INGREDIENTS

- 15 oz. can lentils

- 1 1/2 cups cherry tomato

- 1/4 cup white wine vinegar (or white balsamic vinegar)

- 1/8 cup chives (optional)

- Salt to taste

- Optional additions: olive oil, basil, parsley, etc..

INSTRUCTIONS

- Rinse and drain lentils.

- Add all ingredients and toss to blend. Salt to taste,

if needed, and then fix vinegar.

- Serve immediately or refrigerate in a covered container to allow flavors to develop.

Charred Lettuce And Farro Salad With Salmon

With more fiber per serving than rice, farro is a pantry must-have. This recipe does need it to soak overnight but it is so well worth it. Pile it on a bed of spinach, top with salmon, and then sprinkle with sesame seeds for a lunch that yells the"salad rabbit food" stereotype from the window.

Ingredients

- 1 cup tender farro soaked overnight

- 6 big spinach leaves stalks removed, torn into 1-inch bits

- 1/2 onion chopped

- 1/4 cup pumpkin seeds

- 1/2 cup shaved parmesan

- 2 salmon fillets 6-8 ounce each

- Olive oil

- Salt and pepper to taste

- For the dressing: 2 tablespoon olive oil 2

tablespoons lemon juice, 1 teaspoon garlic clove, 1/4 salt, 1/4 tsp pepper

- Lemon wedges discretionary

Instructions

*The afternoon before, Put 1 cup of sterile farro at a huge bowl, then cover with water (or kefir whey) and let sit at room temperature or in the refrigerator overnight, for 12 or more hrs. Prep time doesn't include soaking.

- If you'd like off soaking liquid strain, it is possible to rinse farro.

- Farro soaked pan, add sufficient water to cover by 1 inch.

- Farro to a boil over medium - heat. When it boils, reduce heat and simmer for 20 minutes.

- Preheat oven Even though the farro is cooking.

- Place salmon on a baking sheet, drizzle with olive oil, salt, and pepper.

- As it flakes with a fork, salmon for 6-10 minutes,

according to the thickness of the fillets, salmon is completed.

- Heat 1 tablespoon of olive oil above medium-high heat in a large skillet.

- Working in batches, place the lettuce, and let sit for 2-3 minutes, until it begins to char.

- Repeat with the kale, adding more olive oil. Set charred kale.

- Place onion slices in skillet and let sit for 2-3 minutes.

- Toss kale, pumpkin seeds, charred onion, cooked farro at a large bowl, and parmesan.

- To prepare dressing, whisk olive oil, lemon juice, minced garlic, and pepper and salt together in a bowl.

- Drizzle salad dressing over salad.

- Top with salmon if desired, and serve with lemon wedges.

Spiced Raisin And Walnut Nut Salad

This salad carries the road less traveled in several ways: by the barley foundation to the mixture of cinnamon, powder, and turmeric. In your hurry to get the doorway, do not rely on the spices outside -- they easy to discover, plus they make all of the difference.

Ingredients:

- 1 cup dry fast cooking starch (or other whole grain)

- 1 cup vegetable broth

- 1 cup water

- 1 Tbsp. Olive oil

- 1 to 2 tsp garlic, minced

- 1 bell pepper, diced

- 1 (15.5 ounce) can navy beans, drained and rinsed

- 1/4 cup raisins (or dried cranberries)

- 1/4 cup pine nuts

- 1/2 tsp. ground turmeric

- **1/4 tsp. All:** cumin, ginger, cinnamon, curry powder, black pepper

- Hot sauce to taste!

Instructions:

- In a medium-sized pot, add barley (or brownish rice/couscous), vegetable broth, and water.

- Bring to a boil, then reduce to a simmer, cover, and cook about 20 minutes, stirring until all liquid has been absorbed and the barley is still fluffy.

- Add the ingredients or stir fry pan. Stir ingredients together over medium heat for approximately 3 minutes, and then add the cooked starch.

- Stir until blended. Warm as is with fresh greens; high with sauce yogurt, if desired.

Healthy Chicken Chickpea Sliced Salad

It is all about flavors and textures in this recipe. Jazz up your chicken salad by pitching in organic sweetness out of corn, some chickpeas to get protein, along with a snack from the goat cheese.

Ingredients

- 2 big romaine hearts, chopped and washed

- 1 cup extracted chicken breast

- 1 (15.5 ounce) can chickpeas, rinsed and drained

- 1 cup grape tomatoes, chopped in half

- 3/4 cup candy corn (I grilled mine)

- 1/4 cup crumbled goat cheese

- 1/3 cup cilantro, chopped and washed

- 1 small avocado, diced

- 1/2 cup BBQ dressing, if desired

Instructions

- Add top with ingredients except BBQ dressing

along with avocado, carrot. Toss salad.

- Put into salad bowls. Garnish with avocado if desired, and garnish with BBQ dressing. Serve with corn tortilla strips that are low carb.

Recipe Notes

- To create vegan omit goat and poultry cheese. Add leafy diced peppers to get taste.

- You may you some dressing you enjoy. I discover I do not need any dressing and enjoy adding two teaspoons of lemon juice.

Marinated Tempeh Salad

Between vegetables, sweet potato, and the tempeh, there is Fiber here for approximately half! Not too shabby for 1 meal. However, so far as flavor is concerned, it is all about the tahini marinade. Permit your tempeh to soak it in as long as you can before grilling to get maximum taste.

INGREDIENTS

- Tempeh - Organic cube (cubed and marinated for 15-20 mins)

- 1-2 Enormous Orange Sweet Potato - Cut to processors and roasted

- 1/2 Red Onion - Finely Sliced

- 1/2 Red Capsicum - Sliced

- Baby Spinach

- Coconut Oil - For Frying

- Paprika

- Salt and Pepper

- MARINADE

- 3 TBS Tahini (Sesame seed paste)

- 1 TBS Tamari (Soy sauce choice)

- 1 Tsp Grated Ginger (finely grated from refreshing)

- 1/2 Lemon - Taste

INSTRUCTIONS

- Preheat oven to 180C

- Clean and prep your potato chips, and then pop them onto a baking tray with pepper, paprika, salt, and a little olive oil. Roast until brown and cooked through.

- Create your curry sauce by mixing well and adding all ingredients.

Dice your tempeh block put into a shallow tray and then coat with the marinade. Put aside for 15-20mins.

- Chop bell pepper and your onion. Rinse the baby and wash spinach.

165

- Add some coconut oil and as soon as the tempeh is prepared, fry until golden brown and cooked through - approx 2mins on each side, based on your cooker temperature.

- After all is cooked, put aside, cooking the diced onion, and including some oil. After your chips have become nice and crispy, remove and you may consume.

- Layout the baby spinach, including the onion cubes, red pepper, and eventually the potato chips.

- Salt and pepper if you want, and love!

NOTES

- A potato can be added by you if functioning two.

- Don't forget to combine the curry it appears to get split and appears strange at first, but as soon as you mix it becomes a paste.

Zucchini Noodle Caprese Salad

Chickpeas provide oomph into the mozzarella and tomato combo To ensure it is a meal using a little protein. With the zoodles in its foundation, it likes eating a bowl of pasta.

INGREDIENTS

- 1 can organic chickpeas (also 1/2 tsp each onion and garlic powder)

- 2 moderate organic zucchini spiralized utilizing blade C

- 2 medium organic vine tomatoes chopped

- 11/2 cups diced fresh mozzarella

- Handful of basil chiffonade

- Balsamic Vinaigrette

- 1 tbsp dijon mustard

- 2 tbsp balsamic vinegar

- 1/4 cup extra virgin olive oil

- Dash of salt

INSTRUCTIONS

- Rinse and drain the chickpeas. You can eat them raw or throw them in a nonstick pan onion and garlic powder and toast with a drizzle of olive oil or spray low for 3 - 5 minutes.

- Dry and spiralize that the zucchini. Squeeze the water from the zucchini using your palms, kitchen towel, or cheesecloth.

- Rinse, dry, and chop the tomatoes. Chop the mozzarella.

- Chop basil.

- For your dressing whisk all of the ingredients.

High Fiber Foods With Wraps And Sandwiches

Dark Bean Avocado Carrot Salad Sandwiches

Forgot to pack lunch before but do not want To hotel to takeout? Been there. Here is something which you may pull together 5 minutes without skimping on taste or nutrition, before leaving. Pack your bread or bread individually.

Ingredients

- 1/2 large avocado, mashed

- 1 may Genova Yellowfin Tuna in olive oil, drained

- 1/2 cup black beans (salt-free or low sodium, favored)

- 1/4 cup chopped cilantro

- 10 grape tomatoes, halved

- Juice out of 1/2 lemon (a lime will even work)

- 1/4 tsp salt

- Freshly ground black pepper, to taste

- 2 slices sprouted, gluten-free or whole-grain bread

(may also use lettuce wraps)

- 2 tablespoons goat cheese crumbles

Instructions

- In a large bowl, mash avocado. Fold in lettuce add the following: cilantro, tomato wedges, lime/lemon juice, pepper, and salt. Mix to blend.

- Bread and spoon lettuce salad at the top. Garnish with goat cheese and cilantro. Enjoy! Makes two open-faced sandwiches.

Turkey Tortilla Wrap With Avocado Cream

These wraps are made healthier by the exchange of the Yogurt spread rather than regular mayo. Along with also the filling of turkey, lettuce and berries can require you back. Ah, easier times.

Ingredients

- 1/2 ripe avocado

- 2-3 tbsp plain Greek yogurt

- 2 tsp fresh lemon juice

- A pinch of pepper and salt

- 2 sprouted whole fermented or grain tortillas

- 4 oz sliced deli-style turkey nitrate-free

- 1 big or two small Roma tomatoes thinly sliced crosswise

- Two handfuls dark lettuce, raw spinach or kale leaves

Instructions

- In a food processor, puree the lemon, lemon juice, salt,

and pepper. Blend the avocado, if you do not have a food processor and combine until creamy and smooth with the yogurt. Put aside.

- Lay 1 tortilla on a flat surface, spread with avocado cream. Roll. Cut around on the diagonal and serve or wrap in parchment or plastic for transportation. Maintain chilled in an ice chest or refrigerated. Eat inside a couple of hours or they might get a bit soggy.

Roasted Red Pepper, Carrot, And Hummus Sandwich

Something simple such as changing from sliced Bread into a baguette can make your sandwich that is normally a lot. Slather using a hummus that is sriracha-spiced, heap in your favorite vegetables, and dig.

INGREDIENTS

- 1 whole-grain sandwich-sized bread loaf or demi-baguette

- 1/2 tsp olive oil

- 1/2 a little avocado

- Salt & pepper

- Pinch red chili pepper flakes, (optional)

- Lemon wedge

- 1/4 cup plain hummus

- 1 tsp sriracha sauce

- 1 large carrot, peeled and chopped into matchsticks

- 2 leaves lacinato kale, ribs removed and finely

chopped

- 1/2 cup loosely packed fire-roasted red peppers

- 1/2 a little cucumber, thinly chopped

INSTRUCTIONS

- Slice the baguette in half lengthwise and scoop bread out of half making sure to leave no less than a 1/4 inch edge of bread and crust. Drizzle both sides with olive oil and toast.

- Mash the avocado. Squeeze the lemon wedge and sprinkle with pepper, salt, and red chili pepper flakes.

- Spoon hummus dispersing it. Sriracha sauce with red peppers, kale, carrots, and cucumbers on hummus and coating. Cover with top of loaf, revel in, and slice in half.

- Nutritional Information is a quote of this sandwich for 1/2.

Chickpea Salad Packs

To get a meal at packaging Lettuce leaves or collard greens instead of pops or bread is an excellent alternative. Here, they which mean you're going to be full even.

Ingredients

- 2 cups cooked chickpeas, drained (if using canned, rinse them well)

- 2 cups baby lettuce, sliced

- 1/4 cup finely chopped red onion

- Juice from 1 large lemon

- 3/4 cup fresh cilantro, sliced

- 1 Tbs. Dijon mustard

- 1 garlic clove, minced

- 1 tsp. ground cumin

- 1/4 tsp smoked paprika

- Freshly ground pepper

- Substantial lettuce or collard green leaves (if

using collard greens, then select smaller sized foliage)

Instructions

- Combine the chickpeas, spinach, and onion into a large bowl.

- In another bowl, whisk together the lemon juice, cilantro, garlic, mustard, cumin, and paprika until well blended.

- Pour along with the chickpea mixture and stir well. Add pepper to taste. Allow the salad marinate.

- Put collard leaves flat on a cutting board (so the stem is pointing up) and carefully shave the length of the stem using a paring knife (being careful to not cut through the foliage). Repeat for every leaf.

- Place leaves cut down and scoop a few of those filling in a vertical column (going the same way as the stem) on a single side Of the foliage. Twist the bottom and top flaps of the foliage toward the middle. Beginning from the side together with all the filling roll from 1 side to the other. If desired, slice in half. Enjoy!

Grilled Vegetable Wrap With Hummus

The veggie wrap is an Entire lunchtime staple, however, Restaurant variations include far tortillas that are bigger and far petroleum than required. This one uses tortillas for a lunch meal which goes easier but still manages to pack in each serving, hummus for taste, and a bit of olive oil.

Ingredients

- 1 12 oz eggplant

- 1 large zucchini

- 1 red bell pepper

- 2 tablespoons + 2 teaspoons olive oil

- 1/2 teaspoon salt

- 1/2 teaspoon ground pepper

- 3/4 tsp ground dried rosemary

- 1/4 cup hummus

- 4 whole-wheat tortillas

- 6 large basil leaves finely chopped

Instructions

- Preheat the grill to medium heat.

- Cut the eggplant to 1/2-inch pieces (complete 12 pieces). Cut the zucchini in half crosswise. Cut each half to 1/4/-inch pieces (complete 8 pieces).

- Lay the zucchini and eggplant slices. Brush with pepper and salt.

- Grill till the vegetables are tender, but not overcooked, about 4 minutes each side for your eggplant and 3 minutes each side for those zucchini and bell pepper.

- Transfer the vegetables to a cutting board and cut them into pieces.

- Spread 1 tbsp on every whole wheat tortilla and split the vegetables and basil leaves.

- Fold the bottom of the tortilla up and fold in the sides. Serve.

Mediterranean Grilled Chicken Wrap

Simple, simple, and satisfying: This Mediterranean Recipe is the best weekday dinner, covering foundations in one bundle. Don't hesitate to use your favorite selection, Although this blogger requires hummus.

Ingredients

- 1 1/4 - 1 1/2 lbs Nature's Promise Chicken Tenders

- 1 tbs olive oil

- 6 Nature's Promise Whole Wheat Tortilla Wraps

- 8 oz. A container of Nature's Promise Roasted Garlic Hummus

- Nature's Promise Baby Spinach

- 1 tbsp dic

- Nature's Promise Grape Tomatoes chopped

- crumbled Feta cheese

Spice Blend

- 1/2 tsp peppermint

- 1/2 tsp paprika

- 1/4 tsp nutmeg

- 1/4 tsp sea salt

- 1/8 tsp garlic powder

Instructions

- Preheat grill to medium (350-400 degrees). Mix the spice mix. Put chicken tenders at a huge bowl, then add oil while blending scatter on the spices so that they coat evenly. Grill until cooked through.

- Distribute a few tablespoons of hummus on each tortilla wrap. Put a few chicken on each and several spinach, then top with the lemon, tomato, and feta. Then roll.

Green Goddess Sandwiches

We can not think of a better title for this particular recipe Four of its seven chief components are green. With avocado, cucumbers, and carrots tucked between thick slices of multigrain bread, then this can be just one unforgettable vegetarian sandwich.

INGREDIENTS

- 2 tsp (ripe)

- 1 teaspoon fresh lemon juice

- Salt and pepper, to taste

- Baby spinach

- 1/4 cup goat cheese (crumbled)

- Freshly ground pepper

- New chives, diced

- Thinly sliced cucumber

- Sprouts (pea, sunflower, alfalfa, etc..)

- 2 pieces Thick of grainy bread, toasted

INSTRUCTIONS

- Get avocado by cutting, eliminating pit, and scooping pulp into a little bowl. Mash with a fork until just lightly. Add salt and lemon juice and pepper, to taste.

- Ready the goat cheese by including a fantastic amount of freshly ground pepper into the goat cheese.

- Toast bread. Once toasted, butter slices and add a little bit of grainy or Dijon mustard to a single piece of every sandwich. The chopped using a coating of baby lettuce. Top the spinach using a coating of the avocado. Goat cheese crumbled. Top the goat cheese with chives. Insert a layer of lemon and top with a layer of sprouts. Add a piece of bread. Press down to compress and cut in half diagonally.

Turkey, Apple, And Brie Sandwich With Apple Cider Mayo

Crisp apples, soft brie, chopped meat, and crusty French bread -- that is a cheese dish at sandwich form. Pack in a fantastic number of arugula for a few additional fiber, and you have got yourself a lunch which you will be tempted to dig way.

Ingredients

- 1 loaf good quality, pre-sliced skillet bread

- 3--4 granny smith apples

- 1 8oz package of Brie cheese, sliced into thin strips (I love to take out the rind that's on top and underside of this cheese, so that you are not getting a lot of it. This way the rind Is Only Going to be around the border)

- 1/2 cm thick-cut turkey breast (new from the deli counter)

- 2 tbsp apple cider vinegar

- 6 tbsp mayonnaise

- Arugula

Instructions

- Toast your pieces of bread lightly from the toaster

- Slice your granny smith apples, and then place aside

- In a small bowl, stir together the carrot and apple cider vinegar

- To assemble the sandwich, then spread around a tablespoon of mayo (less or more depending on taste) onto a piece of bread, add your pieces of brie, your turkey, along with your apples. Finish with a few arugula along with the top piece of bread

High Fiber Recipes For Chief Entrées

Dark Beans And Cauliflower Rice

Create by pulsing it 1 head of cauliflower go a long way Into a foundation for this spin on rice and beans. With a little bit of veggies, a few spices that are Mexican, and sautéing, it's going be tough to discern the difference between the restaurant version.

Ingredients

- 1 can (approximately 15.5 oz) black beans (rinsed and drained)

- 1 large head cauliflower (3 curved cups riced)

- 2 tbsp olive oil

- 3 cloves fresh garlic (minced)

- 1/2 cup fresh sweet onion (finely chopped)

- 1/2 cup fresh red bell pepper (diced)

- 1/4 teaspoon ground cayenne pepper (more or less to taste)

- 3 tbsp pickled jalapeno slices (finely chopped)

- Sea salt and black pepper (to taste)

- 1/2 cup fresh parsley diced (or pops)

Instructions

- Rinse and drain beans. Place on paper towels or even surface for staying water to vanish while preparing the vegetables.

- Cut cauliflower into florets and take out the thick heart. Pulse in smallish batches in food processor to create"rice". See picture in place for consistency. Empty into repeat and then bowl. Whether there are parts of the center, eliminate and discard. A box grater may be utilized as an alternate. You'll need about 3 complete curved cups of cauliflower "rice". Put aside.

- Begin heating olive oil. Add garlic into olive oil and simmer. Add bell pepper, onion, cayenne pepper, salt, and pepper into garlic, stirring, and keep sautéing until onion starts to turn translucent. Add jalapeno and stir fry. Pour cauliflower in addition to vegetables, sprinkle with pepper and salt blend. Keep on cooking approx. 5-7 minutes (until cauliflower is tender but not mushy) stirring and turning around halfway through. Add black beans and cook an additional 2 minutes (sufficient to heat and lightly soften legumes). Add parsley, mix well and serve.

The Very Best Avocado Pasta

If you would like to heat this pasta microwave, but rest assured it is cold. Due to plenty of lemon juice, the meal does not feel heavy, although the avocado sauce is abundant.

Ingredients

- 2 cup raw dry pasta any kind

- 1 ripe avocado halved, seeded and peeled

- 1/4 cup olive oil

- 1/4 cup grated parmesan or romano cheese

- 1/4 cup fresh basil leaves or/and cilantro or parsley I used basil and cilantro and it was wonderful!

- 2 tsp garlic

- 2 tbsp lime or lemon juice

- Salt and freshly ground black pepper to taste

Instructions

- Cook in line with your bundle. Drain well.

- While the pasta is cooking, put the avocado, olive oil, parmesan cheese, garlic, cilantro, and lime juice in a blender or food processor and combine. You procedure it until it is creamy or can make it.

- Toss the pasta with the sauce. Season with pepper and salt to taste and top with romano or parmesan cheese, if desired. Enjoy!

CHAPTER 10
HIGH-FIBER RECIPES FOR
DINNER

High-Fiber Dinners That Are Delicious

Beef And Lentil Stew

S upplying of your Everyday fiber needs lentils are a Delicious way gets sufficient of this nutrient that is digestion-friendly.

Beef Lentil Stew Ingredients

- **Olive Oil --** To saute the garlic, onions, and steak.

- **Steak Chuck --** A fantastic stew meat for taste and texture.

- **Onion --** For depth of taste.

- **Garlic --** For depth of taste.

- **Carrots --** to add sweetness and color.

- **Celery --** to provide feel and herby character.

- **Dried Lentils --** Use green or brown peas, since they maintain their shape after cooking.

- **Crushed Tomatoes --** For sweet taste and thickening.

- **Steak Stock --** To intensify the beefy taste.

- **Red Wine --** To balance the heavy ingredients.

- **Bay Leaves --** To provide profound herby notes.

- **Thyme --** you may use dried or fresh thyme.

- **Cayenne Pepper --** To get just a little kick!

- **Tarragon --** To offer you an original pop of sweetness in the end.

How To Make Beef And Lentil Stew

- Sauté. Heat the oil in a big pot. Sauté the onions then add garlic and the beef.

- Brown. Brown the meat, stirring until the bits are caramelized on either side.

- Dump. Add the celery, carrots, lentils,

tomatoes, beef stock, wine, bay leaves, thyme, 1 tsp salt, and pepper.

- Simmer. Bring to a boil then reduce heat and simmer, until the lentils are tender. Stir in the tarragon!

Lentil Quinoa Meatballs

These meatballs that are lentil are tender the Inside, company on the exterior, and packed with taste that is so much! This is going to be your vegan meatball recipe that is brand new! Love these vegan meatballs having a bowl of spaghetti for the greatest comfort food meal!

Ingredients

- 3 cups water

- 1/4 cup uncooked quinoa rinsed & drained

- 3/4 cup raw french lentils rinsed & drained

- 5-ounce cremini mushrooms (about 5 large mushrooms)

- 1 cup red onion diced (just one little onion)

- 1 cup fermented old fashioned oats (or fermented bread wedges)

- 1 tablespoon ground flaxseed

- 3 tablespoons water

- 1/4 cup sunflower seeds soil

- 2 tablespoon tomato paste

- 1 tablespoon vegan Worcestershire sauce

- 2 tablespoons nutritional yeast

- 2 garlic cloves minced (or 1 teaspoon garlic powder)

- 1 tablespoon Italian seasonings

- 1 teaspoon dried basil

- 1 teaspoon dried parsley

- 1/2 tsp sour pink sea salt to taste

- 1/4 teaspoon black pepper

Instructions

- Begin with boiling 3 cups of water. After the water boils, season it with salt and include 3/4 cup of raw lentils that are drained and rinsed. Reduce the heat and set a timer for 24 minutes.

- Insert 1/4 cup of quinoa whenever there are 12 minutes left on the timer and stir it. Allow the peas and quinoa continues cooking together till there's not any water. It ought to take a total of 23-24 minutes to cook quinoa and the lentils.

- Allow the cooked quinoa mixture cool for a couple of minutes. Add 3 tablespoons of water and 1 tablespoon of ground flaxseed into a bowl, while it's cooling. Mix it and place it in the refrigerator.

- Use a coffee grinder or cup that is little to grind sunflower seeds.

- Pour the peas and quinoa to a massive food processor (that is the 13 cup food processor that I use and enjoy!). Add the roughly chopped cremini mushrooms, diced red onion, old fashioned oats, mixed sunflower seeds, tomato paste, vegan Worcestershire sauce, nutritional yeast, Italian seasonings, garlic powder, dried basil, dried parsley, pepper, salt, and the egg.

- The filling united and high for 1-2 minutes or till of the ingredients have been broken down. The mixture will be sticky but that is normal.

(A moist batter leaves moist lentil meatballs, a sterile batter could lead to dry vegan meatballs.)

- Preheat the oven to 350 degrees.

- Line a baking dish while the oven is warming. Use an ice cream scoop or large spoon to scoop the filling from the food processor and use your hands to roll up the filling into golfing vegan meatballs. Vegan meatballs will be made by the filling.

- Organize the vegan meatballs on the menu and inhale them. Drink the hot lentil meatballs with tomato sauce, a sprinkle of nutrient yeast (or vegan parm), and serve the meatballs on your favorite pasta.

Steak And Broccoli

Broccoli and beef is a dish you'll find in Takeout or all restaurant areas. I like broccoli and beef because (a) I cannot resist anything with yummy and tender pieces of flank steak, and (b) it is such a simple one-pan stir fry recipe that requires less than 30 minutes total. If you are a broccoli lover like me, you will love these yummy and hot snacks of broccoli between mouthfuls of rice and beef.

Ingredients

- 1 lb flank steak sliced into 1/4 inch thick bits

- 3 cups small broccoli florets

- 1/2 cup beef stock

- 5 cloves garlic minced

- 2 tbsp corn starch

- 1 tbsp canola oil

For the sauce:

- 1/2 cup low sodium soy sauce

- 1/4 cup brown sugar

- 2 tsp corn starch

INSTRUCTIONS

- Toss chopped steak with corn starch in a large bowl.

- Heat canola oil in a pan over moderate heat. Add steak and cook until it browns, a couple of minutes, stirring. Transfer to a plate and set aside.

- Add garlic and broccoli and stir fry. Add meats. Let simmer until the broccoli is tender, approximately 10 minutes, stirring periodically.

- While awaiting the broccoli combine all the sauce ingredients and combine well.

- Add sauce and the beef and stir fry. Let simmer.

- Serve broccoli and steak.

Yellow Lentil Curry

This simple and flavorful yellow dal is filled with protein and vivid flavors! It is great by itself or served to get a mid-week meal that is healthful and fast!

Ingredients

- 2 tbsp olive or coconut oil

- 1 large onion diced finely

- 1 Thai chili diced finely

- 4 garlic cloves minced onto a Microplane

- 2 tbsp ginger grated onto a Microplane

- 1.5 cups

- 1 tablespoon ground turmeric

- 2 tsp curry powder

- 1 teaspoon garam masala

- 3-4 cups low-sodium vegetable broth

- 1 can diced tomatoes

- Juice of half a lime

- Salt and ground black pepper to taste

- Cilantro to garnish

- Lime wedges to garnish

- Cooked basmati rice

Instructions

- Add oil.

- Add chilies, garlic, ginger, and onions and let you sweat over moderate heat. Don't permit any color.

- Add spices, lentils, tomatoes, 2 cups of broth, and season with pepper and salt.

- Bring to a simmer and reduce to low. Cook using a lid opens for 20 minutes. Stir often also to check for fluid and to prevent burning the ground. The liquid add more broth when the lentils have consumed. You desire this thick but still have loads of liquid.

- After the lentils have attained the desired doneness and feel adjust for seasoning and heat and add lime juice and serve on rice.

- Garnish with cilantro

Chickpea Broccoli Buddha Bowl

This Chickpea Broccoli Buddha Bowl is a meal with roasted veggies, plant protein, plus a sauce. Perfect for children and adults alike!

Ingredients

For your bowls:

- 1--15oz can chickpeas, drained and rinsed

- 2 heads broccoli, chopped into florets

- 3 medium carrots, sliced (1 teaspoon cup)

- 1 tablespoon extra virgin olive oil

- Salt and freshly ground black pepper, to taste

- 2 cups cooked brown rice or quinoa

For the sauce:

- 1/4 cup organic creamy peanut butter

- 1/4 cup vanilla milk (more if necessary to lean)

- 1 tbsp + 1 tsp reduced-sodium soy sauce (sub

tamari for gluten-free)

- 1 tbsp + 1 teaspoon pure maple syrup

- splash of lime juice or rice vinegar (optional)

- 1 teaspoon minced ginger (optional) plus a pinch red pepper flakes (optional)

Instructions

- Preheat oven to 400F. Line a baking sheet using a parchment or Silpat paper. Put chickpeas, broccoli, and carrots on the baking sheet.

- Roast for 20-25 minutes, stirring halfway through.

- Cook. I used frozen rice, making it simple!

- Put peanut butter in a medium bowl and microwave for around 20 minutes (optional, but that can make it much easier to stir fry). Add red pepper flakes, soy sauce, maple syrup, ginger, and milk and whisk till smooth.

- Collect dishes by putting grains in the base

topped with a good deal and mix of peanut sauce.

Turmeric Chickpea Salad Sandwich

Searching for a vegetarian sandwich recipe? Try out this turmeric chickpea salad! It is filled with taste and protein -- also an alternative into egg salad sandwich or some tuna salad! Insert devour and your sandwich toppings.

Ingredients

- 1 can chickpeas - emptied

- 1/3 cup aquafaba or vegan mayo*

- 1/2 tsp garlic

- 1/2 tsp onion powder

- 1 tsp garlic - minced

- Black pepper to taste

- Salt to taste

Instructions

- Pulse all ingredients in a blender and cracked down, but not entirely mushy. You need some feel in there!

- Ground Turkey Sweet Potato Skillet

- This Universe Turkey Sweet Potato Skillet is going to be ready to consume And you'll be astounded by flavorful it's. It is a meal for the family!

Ingredients

- 2 tbsp extra virgin olive oil

- 1 lb free-range extra-lean ground turkey -- (you can utilize grass-fed ground beef)

- 1 tsp garlic clove -- minced

- 1/2 cup onions -- diced

- 1/2 cup yellow pepper diced

- 11/2 cups sweet potato -- diced

- Salt and freshly ground black pepper

- A pinch of red chili flakes -- optional

- 1/2 cup shredded mozzarella cheese (In case you are doing Whole30 or after Paleo diet, then do not add cheese)

- Fresh parsley -- for garnishing (optional)

Instructions

- On medium-high heat, heat the oil in a cast-iron skillet.

- Add the ground garlic and turkey. Use a wooden spoon as it cooks. Stir and cook for approximately 5 minutes.

- Add peppers and the onions, and cook till the onions are tender.

- Add pepper, red chili flakes, salt, and the potato.

- Cover and cook till the potatoes are tender. Do not forget to stir. Add a tiny bit of water or more olive oil to cook the potatoes.

- Preheat the oven while the potatoes are cooking.

- When the potatoes are tender, then add the mozzarella cheese, and set the skillet in the oven.

- Remove from the oven when the cheese melts

and garnish with parsley.

- Sweet Potato and Avocado Burger

- Homemade Sweet Potato Burgers -- healthful and tasty!

Ingredients

- 1 medium sweet potato

- 1 1/2 cups drained and rinsed canned cannellini beans

- 2-3 tablespoon oat or wheat germ

- 1 tablespoon tahini or nut butter, softened

- 1 teaspoon pure maple syrup, or pinch stevia for sugar-free

- 1/4 tsp garlic powder or spice mix

- Salt, pepper, optional cayenne or other spices

- Optional 1-2 tablespoons nutritional yeast

- If skillet: 1-3 teaspoon vegetable or coconut oil

- Optional 1/2 cup panko breadcrumbs or 1/4

cup cooked brown rice

- Toppings of selection

Instructions

Preheat oven a couple holes in the potato A fork. Bake until extremely and sticky-sweet tender. Remove and set the curry's flesh in a huge bowl. Add tahini, flour, beans, maple syrup, spices, and seasonings and then use a fork. Cover and refrigerate until the mixture is firm enough to readily manage (15-20 minutes). The mixture will be moist and soft, therefore add the additional flour as necessary (or fold into 1/4 cup into 1/2 cup breadcrumbs) till it's possible to form patties. *If skillet Heat 1 tablespoon oil on high heat at a pan. Coat them with the breadcrumbs and Type 5 patties, then put each side or until browned. Transfer to a paper towel and let cool. *When baking: Omit the coating, and then fold 1/4 cup cooked rice. Bake in 350 F onto a baking sheet for 20 minutes. Burgers will be lightly browned.

Quinoa And Sweet Potato Chili

Try this healthy, vegetarian quinoa chili with luminous sweet Potatoes and potatoes that are hearty. The best part? It is made at a slower cooker, so it is largely hands-off and simple!

Ingredients

- 3 cups diced sweet potato roughly 1 big

- 1 cup diced red onion roughly 1 moderate

- 1 cup diced bell peppers around 1 big

- 3 garlic cloves minced

- 1 15 ounce can black beans

- 1 28 ounce can of flame-roasted tomatoes

- 3 -- 4 cups vegetable broth

- 2 tbsp tomato paste

- 1/2 cup uncooked quinoa

- 1 -- 1 1/2 tablespoons chili powder

- 2 tsp cumin

210

- 2 tsp paprika

- 1 tsp coriander

- 1/2 teaspoon cayenne less or more to taste

- Salt & pepper to taste

Instructions

- Add all ingredients into a crockpot (beginning with only 3 cups of broth). Turn on top and cook for 4 hours, then turn down to low and continue to cook till ready to serve. Stir in a different 1/2 -- 1 cup of water if too thick.

- Serve with diced avocado (or guac) along with tortilla chips). It is such a great combo!

One-Pan Garlic Roasted Salmon And Brussels Sprouts

One Sheet Pan Garlic Roasted Salmon with Brussels sprouts -- Incredibly delicious, garlicky yummy supper together with salmon and brussels sprouts.

Ingredients

FOR THE BRUSSELS SPROUTS

- 2 pounds brussels sprouts, ends trimmed

- 3 tbsp STAR Garlic Flavored Olive Oil

- 1/2 tsp salt

- 1/4 tsp fresh ground pepper

For The Salmon

- 2 pounds salmon fillet, skinned and cut into 6 parts

- 1 tbsp STAR Garlic Flavored Olive Oil

- 3 to 4 garlic cloves, minced

- 1 tbsp dried oregano

212

- 1/2 tsp salt

- Fresh ground pepper, to taste

Instructions

- Preheat oven to 450F.

- Lightly grease a baking sheet and set aside.

- In a large mixing bowl blend brussels sprouts, salt, olive oil, and pepper; combine until blended.

- Transfer brussels sprouts to the baking sheet.

- Meanwhile, prepare the salmon.

- Drizzle salmon.

- Evenly press and split minced garlic.

- Season with salt, oregano, and pepper.

- Remove baking sheet proceed the brussels sprouts about, producing 6 stains.

- Place salmon in spots and then bake for 10 to 12 minutes, or until salmon is cooked through.

- Remove from oven let stand 2 minutes and serve.

Vegan Lentil Sloppy Joe

This Variant of the classic Joes has the same taste. And they are a breeze. Toss everything and allow it to do the job for you!

Ingredients

- 1 cup finely chopped carrots

- 1 cup finely sliced mushrooms

- 1 cup thinly sliced onions

- 2 garlic cloves minced

- 1 1/2 cups

- 1/2 cup quinoa

- 1 8oz can tomato sauce

- 1/2 cup organic ketchup I used agave sweetened

- 2 tbsp maple syrup

- 2 tbsp hot sauce

- 2 tbsp mustard

- 1 tbsp chili powder

- 1 tsp paprika

- Pinch of pepper & salt

- 3 - 4 cups vegetable broth

Instructions

- Insert everything to the slow cooker. Stir to blend, cover, and set to high. Cook on high for 2 - 3 hours (or low for 4 - 6). Assess and add liquid.

- Serve warm inside a skillet or biscuit, with a bun!

Beet, Edamame, and Quinoa Salad

Reset with this beet salad recipe Superfoods such as edamame, quinoa, spinach, lettuce, and avocado. It is as colorful as it's healthy! Steak yields four side salads or two salads. If you anticipate having leftovers, then keep the greens from the ingredients that are ready and toss before serving.

Ingredients

- Salad

- 1/2 cup uncooked quinoa, rinsed

- 1 cup frozen organic edamame

- 1/3 cup slivered almonds or pepitas (green pumpkin seeds)

- 1 medium raw beet, peeled

- 1 medium-to-large carrot (or 1 extra moderate beet), peeled

- 2 cups packed baby spinach or arugula, roughly sliced

- 1 avocado, cubed

Vinaigrette

- 3 tbsp apple cider vinegar

- 2 tbsp lime juice

- 2 tbsp olive oil

- 1 tbsp chopped fresh mint or cilantro

- 2 tbsp honey or maple syrup or agave nectar

- 1/2 to 1 tsp Dijon mustard, to taste

- 1/4 tsp salt

- Freshly ground black pepper, to taste

Instructions

- To cook the quinoa: First, rinse the quinoa in a fine mesh colander under running water for 2 or a moment. In a pot, mix one cup water and the quinoa. Bring the mixture to a boil, then cover the pot, reduce heat, and cook for 15 minutes. Eliminate from heat and let it break for 5 minutes. Uncover the pot, drain any excess water off, and dab on the quinoa. Set it aside to cool.

- To cook then add the edamame and cook until the beans are heated through, about 5 minutes. Drain and put aside.

- To pepitas or toast the almonds: In a skillet over moderate heat, toast pepitas or the almonds, stirring regularly, until they are aromatic and beginning to turn golden on the edges. Transfer into a serving bowl to cool.

- To ready the beet(s) or carrot: First of all, don't hesitate to simply chop them finely as possible with a sharp chef's knife OR grate them on a box grater. In case you've got a spiralizer, then you can spiralize C being used by them dip the ribbons into little pieces. In case you've got a mandoline and julienne peeler (this is a nuisance), utilize the mandoline into julienne the beet and utilize a julienne peeler into julienne the carrot then dip the ribbons into little pieces with a sharp chef's knife.

- To prepare the vinaigrette: Whisk together all the ingredients until emulsified.

- To assemble the salad: In your big serving bowl, combine the toasted almonds/pepitas, cooked edamame, ready beet(s), and/or lettuce, roughly chopped spinach/arugula (see note above leftovers), cubed avocado and cooked quinoa.

- Ultimately, drizzle dressing over the mix (you may not need it all) and lightly toss to combine. Should you throw it 14, you are going to get a salad! Season to taste with salt (up to an extra 1/4 tsp) and black pepper. Serve.

Spicy Kimchi Quinoa Bowl

These kimchi quinoa bowls are the ideal weeknight dinner. They are simple and super fast healthy, packed with protein, fermented vegetables, and greens!

Ingredients

- 2 tsp toasted sesame oil

- 1/2 tsp freshly grated ginger

- 1 tsp minced garlic

- 2 cups cooked quinoa chilled

- 1 cup kimchi chopped

- 2 tsp kimchi"juice" the liquid out of the jar

- 2 tsp fermented tamari

- 1 tsp hot sauce discretionary

- 2 cups spinach finely chopped

- 2 eggs

- 1/4 cup chopped green onions for garnish discretionary

- Fresh ground pepper for garnish discretionary

Instructions

- Heat the oil in a skillet over moderate heat. Add garlic and ginger and simmer for 30 - 60 minutes till aromatic. Add kimchi and the quinoa and cook about 2 - 3 minutes. Stir in tamari, juice, and hot sauce if using. Switch to low as you prepare the other components and stir occasionally.

- In another skillet, cook until the whites have cooked but the yolks are still runny, about 3 - 5 minutes.

- Steam the kale - 60 minutes till tender.

- Collect the dishes, dividing the mix that is kimchi-quinoa and kale between 2 meals. Top with green onions and pepper if

Spinach Pesto Quinoa Bowl

The finest part is, you probably have these ingredients in your cabinet.

Ingredients

- 2 cups multi-colored quinoa, raw

- 6 cups baby spinach

- 4 tbsp basil pesto

- 1/2 tsp kosher salt

- 1/2 cup freshly grated Parmesan cheese and more for topping

Instructions

- Cook quinoa in line with the instructions on the tote or the box. (Rather than plain water, I used chicken stock for more taste but if you would like to maintain this vegetarian dish, proceed with water or vegetable stock.)

- After quinoa is done cooking, then turn heat to medium then add pesto, spinach, salt, and cheese. Stir pesto is dispersed, and Parmesan cheese has melted.

- Serve with additional cheese, if desired.

CHAPTER 11
HIGH-FIBER RECIPES FOR
WEIGHT LOSS

Fiber-Rich Recipes To Help You Shed Weight

Add more fiber to your meal. The Average adult that is American gains one according to reports. But new research indicates a way to avoid this weight reduction or promote weight reduction. The key? Eat more fiber. These recipes allow you to get your fill.

Chicken & White Bean Salad

Celery and zucchini provide a pleasant to this salad crunch. We enjoy serving it on a bed of radicchio and escarole, but any kind of salad greens will probably get the job done.

Ingredients

- Vinaigrette

- 1 medium clove garlic

- 1/4 tsp salt

- 5 tbsp peppermint oil

- 6 tbsp fresh orange juice, plus more to taste

- 1/4 cup white-wine vinegar or red-wine vinegar

- 1 tbsp Dijon mustard

Salad

- 1 15-ounce may cannellini or other white beans, rinsed and drained

- 2 1/2 cups diced cooked chicken breast (see Tips)

- 2 cups diced zucchini or summertime squash (about 2 small)

- 1 1/2 cups diced celery

- 1/4 cup finely diced ricotta Salata, halloumi (see Tips) or feta cheese

- 1/3 cup sliced, well-drained, oil-packed sun-dried tomatoes (optional)

- 1 cup coarsely chopped fresh basil, and whole basil leaves for garnish

- Salt & freshly ground pepper to taste (optional)

- 2 cups torn escarole or romaine lettuce

- 2 cups torn radicchio leaves

Instructions

- To prepare vinaigrette: Peel the garlic and crush together with a chef's knife's aspect. With a fork, mash the tsp salt in a bowl to make a paste. Whisk in 5 tbsp oil. Add juice, mustard, and vinegar. Whisk and taste up to 4 tbsp more juice mellows the taste; year. Set aside at room temperature.

- To prepare salad: Combine beans, chicken, zucchini (or summertime squash), celery, cheese, and sun-dried tomatoes (if using) in a large bowl till well mixed. Add 3/4 cup vinaigrette and ginger; toss until blended. Taste and season with pepper or salt, if desired.

- Toss the rest of the vinaigrette with escarole (or romaine) and radicchio in a skillet. Serve the salad onto the greens, garnished with basil leaves.

Shrimp Panzanella

This fresh-tasting Panzanella (Italian bread-and-tomato Salad) consists of shrimp, olives, and a good deal of herbs. You are going to want olives packed with brine that is yummy to produce the dressing table. Purchase shrimp peeled and cooked. On occasion, the shrimp can be bought frozen. Drink cold water for 10 minutes.

Ingredients

- 4 tbsp extra-virgin olive oil, split

- 1 teaspoon garlic, peeled and halved

- 4 cups 1/2-inch crusty multigrain bread cubes, rather day-old

- 1 lb coarsely chopped peeled cooked shrimp

- 4 large ripe but firm tomatoes, coarsely chopped

- 2 large green, red or yellowish bell peppers, diced

- 3/4 cup chopped fresh parsley

- 1/4 cup sliced fresh chives

- 1/4 cup chopped pitted Kalamata olives, also 1/4

cup olive brine

- 3 tbsp red-wine vinegar

- 1 1/2 tsp chopped fresh coriander or 3/4 tsp dried

- Freshly ground pepper to taste

- 4 cups mixed salad greens

Instructions

- Preheat oven to 350 degrees F.

- Drizzle 2 tablespoons oil onto a rimmed baking sheet. Mash garlic to the oil using a fork to infuse it discard the garlic. Stir bread cubes to the oil until coated. Bake, stirring every 5 minutes, until very sharp, 12 to 15 minutes. Let cool.

- Tomatoes, shrimp, bell peppers, parsley, chives, olives and olive brine, vinegar, thyme, and the remaining 2 tbsp oil in a large bowl... Let stand for 10 or more minutes to blend the flavors.

- Toss serves the salad and the croutons with the shrimp mixture.

228

Creamy Garlic Pasta With Shrimp & Vegetables

Toss a Middle Eastern-inspired that is garlicky chili sauce with Pasta, shrimp, peas, peas, and red bell pepper for a summertime meal that is satisfying. Drink: Slices of tomato and lemon tossed with olive oil and lemon juice.

Ingredients

- 6 oz whole-wheat spaghetti

- 12 oz peeled and deveined raw fish), cut to 1-inch bits

- 1 bunch asparagus, trimmed and thinly sliced

- 1 large red bell pepper, thinly chopped

- 1 cup frozen or fresh peas

- 3 cloves garlic, sliced

- 1 1/4 tsp kosher salt

- 1 1/2 cups nonfat or low-fat yogurt

- 1/4 cup sliced flat-leaf parsley

- 3 tbsp lemon juice

- 1 tbsp peppermint oil

- 1/2 tsp freshly ground pepper

- 1/4 cup toasted pine nuts

Instructions

- Bring a large pot of water. Add spaghetti and cook two minutes less than package instructions. Add asparagus, beans, bell pepper and peas and cook until the pasta is tender and the fish are cooked. Drain well.

- Mash garlic and salt in a bowl before a Glue forms. Whisk in yogurt, parsley, lemon juice, pepper, and oil. Insert the pasta mixture and toss to coat. Serve sprinkled with pine nuts (if using).

Hot Chile Grilled Cheese

This version of a chile Relleno turned Sandwich packs also a filling and some warmth. Any sort of bread will do the job, although we enjoy the taste of sourdough. Drink: pineapple and Coleslaw.

Ingredients

- 4 poblano peppers (see Notice)

- 1 14-ounce may pinto beans, rather low-sodium

- 3 tablespoons prepared salsa

- ⅛ tsp salt

- 1/2 cup shredded Monterey Jack or Cheddar cheese

- 2 tbsp low-fat plain yogurt

- 3 scallions, sliced

- 2 tsp chopped fresh cilantro

- 8 slices sourdough bread

Instructions

- Put peppers in a bowl, then cover with plastic wrap and microwave on High 3 to 4 minutes, until tender. Let stand until cool enough to handle.

- Combine salsa beans and salt. Mash the beans with a fork till they start to produce a paste (some could stay whole). Combine yogurt, cheese, scallions, and cilantro.

- If the peppers are cool enough to handle, slice each one in half lengthwise and remove seeds and the stem.

- Spread 1/3 cup of the bean mixture. Top with a tablespoon. Put two pepper halves over the cheese. Cover with the remaining pieces of bread.

- Grill the sandwiches at the maker until golden brown. Cut in half and serve.

- Stovetop Version: Place 15-ounce cans along with also a medium skillet (not nonstick) from the cooker. Heat 1 tsp olive oil over moderate heat in a nonstick skillet. Place 2 sandwiches in the pan.

Put the medium skillet then weight it down. Cook about two minutes, until golden on one side. Reduce the heat to medium-low, reverse the sandwiches, then replace the skillet and cans, and cook until the second side is golden, 1 to 3 minutes longer. Repeat with the two sandwiches and another 1 tsp oil.

Grilled Fish Tacos

Rather than deep-frying the fish to these fish tacos, Coat the fish and grill it. Be certain that the fillets are not any longer than thick so that they cook. Sometimes fish on the grill can be hard because the fish and the grill could stick together or fall. The remedy would be to purchase a basket that corrects the fish at the basket for easy and holds 4 to 6 fish fillets. If you do not have a grilling basket, then be sure that the grill is warm and nicely oiled before adding fish.

Adobo-Rubbed Fish

- 4 tsp chili powder, preferably created with New Mexico or ancho chiles

- 2 tbsp lime juice

- 2 tbsp peppermint oil

- 1 tsp ground cumin

- 1 tsp onion powder

- 1 tsp garlic powder

- 1 tsp salt

234

- 1/2 tsp freshly ground pepper

- 2 pounds mahi-mahi or Pacific halibut 1/2-3/4 inch thick, skinned and cut into 4 parts

Coleslaw

- 1/4 cup reduced-fat sour cream

- 1/4 cup low-carb snacking

- 2 tbsp chopped fresh cilantro

- 1 tsp lime zest

- 2 tbsp lime juice

- 1 tsp sugar

- ⅛ tsp salt

- Freshly ground pepper

- 3 cups finely shredded green or red cabbage

- 12 corn tortillas, heated

Instructions

- To prepare fish chili powder salt, garlic powder, and pepper in a bowl. Rub adobo rub on over fish.

Let stand 20 to 30 minutes to the fish.

- To prepare coleslaw: Blend sour cream, mayonnaise, cilantro, lime zest, lime juice, sugar, pepper, and salt in a medium bowl mix until creamy and smooth. Add cabbage and toss to blend. Refrigerate till ready to use.

- Preheat grill.

- Oil the grill rack (see Hint) or use a grilling basket. Grill the fish until it's cooked through and easily flakes with a fork. Transfer the fish to a bowl and divide it into chunks.

- Drink the tacos family-style by passing the fish, tortillas, coleslaw, and taco garnishes separately.

Greek Orzo Stuffed Peppers

We steam colored bell peppers at the microwave to Conserve time and stuff them with feta, spinach, and orzo. This recipe may work with just about any filling--attempt substituting several kinds of herbs, cheese, or beans. Serve with pineapple salad and pita bread.

Ingredients

- 4 orange, yellow or reddish bell peppers

- 1/2 cup whole-wheat orzo

- 1 15-ounce can chickpeas, rinsed

- 1 tbsp peppermint oil

- 1 medium onion, chopped

- 6 oz baby spinach, coarsely chopped

- 1 tbsp chopped fresh oregano, or 1 tsp dried

- 3/4 cup crumbled feta cheese, split

- 1/4 cup sun-dried tomatoes, (maybe not oil-packed), sliced

- 1 tbsp sherry vinegar or red-wine vinegar

- 1/4 tsp salt

Instructions

- Halve peppers lengthwise leaving the stalks. Set the peppers cut-side down in a massive dish. Insert 1/2 in. water, then cover and microwave on High until the peppers are just softened, 7 to 9 minutes. Let cool slightly, drain and put aside.

- Bring a large saucepan of water. Add orzo and cook until just tender, 8 to 10 minutes or according to package instructions. Drain and rinse with cold water.

- Mash chickpeas leaving a few whole.

- Heat oil in a nonstick skillet over moderate heat. Add onion and cook for about 4 minutes. Add simmer and spinach and cook, stirring until the spinach is wilted, about 1 minute. Stir in chickpeas the orzo, 1/2 cup feta, tomatoes, salt, and vinegar; cook till heated through, about 1 minute. Divide the filling halves and sprinkle each pepper with a number of the cup feta.

Vegetarian Tortilla Soup

"Tortilla soup includes a location, I believe, in virtually every Collection of Mexican foods," states Rick Bayless. It is a vegetarian version of the soup. Earthy pasilla chile tastes the soul-satisfying broth.

Ingredients

- 3 large dried pasilla (negro), ancho or New Mexico chiles (see Notice)

- 1 15-ounce can diced tomatoes, rather fire-roasted

- 2 tablespoons and 2 teaspoons olive oil or extra-virgin olive oil, split

- 1 medium white onion, sliced 1/4 inch thick

- 3 cloves garlic, peeled

- 4 cups vegetable broth or "no-chicken" broth

- 4 cups water

- 1 large sprig epazote (optional; see Notice)

- 1 14-ounce bundle extra-firm tofu

- 4 cups sliced chard, spinach or kale leaves

- 1/4-1/2 tsp salt

- 1 ripe large avocado, cut into 1/4-inch cubes

- 2 cups about broken tortilla chips

- 3/4 cup shredded Mexican melting cheese, like Chihuahua or asadero, or Monterey Jack or mild Cheddar (discretionary)

- 1 large lime, cut into 6 wedges

Instructions

- Holding the chiles one at a time together with metal tongs, immediately toast them by turning an inch or two over an open fire for several minutes until the aroma fills the kitchen. (Instead, toast chiles in a dry pan over moderate heat, pressing them flat for a couple of seconds then turning them and pressing)

- Break them into pieces when cool enough to handle, stem and seed the chiles and set them in a blender together with their juice and tomatoes. (A food processor will work, even though it will not fully puree the chiles.)

- Heat 2 tbsp oil in a Dutch oven over moderate heat. Add garlic and onion and cook, stirring often, until golden, 6 to 9 minutes. Scoop up garlic and the onion with a slotted spoon and transfer to the blender together with the tomato mix.

- Return the pot to medium heat. When very hot, add the puree and stir fry constantly until thickened to the consistency of tomato paste. Add water, broth and epazote (if using). Bring to a boil, and then adjust heat to maintain a simmer.

- Drain tofu, rinse, and pat cut to cubes - into 1/2. Heat the remaining 2 tsp oil. Cook and add the tofu stirring every 2-3 minutes 6 to 8 minutes total. Add the tofu.

- Add chard (or lettuce or spinach) into the soup and season with salt to taste, depending on the saltiness of the broth. Cook until the greens are wilted, about two minutes, depending on the kind of greens.

- Ladle the soup into 8 soup bowls. Split avocado, tortilla chips, and cheese (if using) one of the bowls. Serve warm, with lime wedges.

Broccoli, Ham & Pasta Salad

This pasta salad, A Excellent entree is loaded with peppers and broccoli. Peppers and ham give lots of punch to it. Appreciate the leftovers to get a lunch.

Ingredients

- 1/2 cup low-carb snacking

- 1/3 cup nonfat plain yogurt

- 1/4 cup reduced-fat sour cream

- 3 tbsp rice vinegar or white-wine vinegar

- 1 tbsp Dijon mustard

- 1 tbsp honey, or more to taste

- 1 1/2 tsp dried minced onion or dried chopped chives

- 1 1/4 tsp dried tarragon or dill

- 1/2 tsp onion salt or celery or 1/4 tsp of every

- White pepper to taste

Salad

- 3 cups cooked whole-wheat fusilli or rice (about 6 oz dry)

- 4 cups chopped broccoli florets (about 1 1/2 big heads)

- 1 1/2 cups diced ham (8 oz), rather reduced-sodium

- 1 large yellow or red bell pepper (or a mix), diced

- 1/4 cup diced red onion, also pieces for garnish

- 1/3 cup raisins

- Freshly ground pepper to taste

- 4 cups spinach leaves

- 1 cup torn radicchio leaves

Instructions

- To prepare dressing: Combine mayonnaise, yogurt, sour cream, vinegar, mustard, honey, onion (or chives), tarragon (or dill), and onion salt (or celery salt) in a bowl till well-mixed taste and adjust seasonings, if desired.

- To prepare salad broccoli, pasta, bell pepper, ham, diced onion, and raisins in a bowl that is. Add dressing and toss until evenly incorporated. Cover and simmer to blend the flavors for as many as 2 days and a minimum of 30 minutes.

- Serve on a bed of radicchio and spinach, garnished with pieces of onion.

Brothy Chinese Noodles

Earth was inspired by Dan Dan noodles -- Noodles and Pork in a hot broth. We omit the Sichuan peppercorns for advantage and use ground turkey, but include hot sesame oil. If you would like noodles to use eucalyptus oil.

Ingredients

- 2 tbsp warm sesame oil (see Notice), split

- 1 pound 93 percent -lean ground turkey

- 1 bunch scallions, chopped, split

- 2 tsp garlic, minced

244

- 1 tbsp minced fresh ginger

- 4 cups reduced-sodium poultry broth

- 3/4 cup water

- 3 cups thinly sliced bok choy

- 8 oz dried Chinese noodles (see Notice)

- 3 tbsp reduced-sodium soy sauce

- 1 tbsp rice vinegar

- 1 small lemon, sliced into matchsticks, for garnish

Instructions

- Heat 1 tbsp oil in a saucepan over moderate heat. Add all but two tbsp of the scallions, ground turkey, garlic and ginger and cook, stirring and breaking up the turkey, about 5 minutes, until no longer pink. Transfer to a plate.

- Add bok choy, water, broth, noodles, soy sauce, vinegar, and the remaining 1 tbsp oil. Bring to a boil. Cook until the noodles are tender. Pour the turkey mixture and stir to blend. Serve garnished with the reserved 2 tbsp scallions and lemon (if using).

Grilled Eggplant & Portobello Sandwich

On the lookout for a vegetarian choice for the next cookout? This Portobello sandwich and Grilled eggplant is our response. We top it with pieces of hot arugula and tomato. Serve with a salad.

Ingredients

- 1 small clove garlic, sliced

- 1/4 cup low-carb snacking

- 1 tsp lemon juice

- 1 medium eggplant (about 1 lb), sliced into 1/2-inch rounds

- 2 large or 3 medium portobello mushroom caps, gills removed (see Hint)

- Canola or olive oil cooking spray

- 1/2 tsp salt

- 1/2 tsp freshly ground pepper

- 8 pieces whole-wheat sandwich bread, gently grilled or toasted

- 2 cups arugula, or spinach, stemmed and sliced if large

- 1 large tomato, sliced

Instructions

- Preheat grill.

- Mash garlic into a paste. Blend with lemon and mayonnaise juice in a small bowl. Put aside.

- Coat both sides of mushroom caps and eggplant rounds with cooking spray and season with pepper and salt. Grill the vegetables, turning once, until tender and browned on both sides: 2 to 3 minutes each side for eggplant. When cool enough to handle, slice the mushrooms.

- Spread 1 1/2 teaspoon of the garlic mayonnaise on each slice of bread. Layer the eggplant, mushrooms, arugula (or lettuce), and tomato pieces onto 4 slices of bread and top with the bread.

Chicken & Spinach Soup with Fresh Pesto

This aromatic soup benefit from Ingredients --skinless chicken breast boneless baby spinach and beans. It sports a homemade basil pesto swirled in at the end. You can substitute 3 to 4 tbsp of pesto if you're very pressed for time.

Ingredients

- 2 teaspoons plus 1 tablespoon extra-virgin olive oil, split

- 1/2 cup lettuce or diced red bell pepper

- 1 large boneless, skinless chicken breast (about 8 ounces), cut into quarters

- 1 large clove garlic, minced

- 5 cups reduced-sodium poultry broth

- 1 1/2 tsp dried marjoram

- 6 oz baby spinach, coarsely chopped

- 1 15-ounce can cannellini beans or great northern beans, rinsed

- 1/4 cup grated Parmesan cheese

- 1/3 cup lightly packed fresh basil leaves

- Freshly ground pepper to taste

- 3/4 cup plain or herbed multigrain croutons for garnish (optional)

Instructions

- Heat 2 tsp oil in a large saucepan or Dutch oven above medium-high heat. Add carrot (or bell pepper) and poultry; cook, turning the fish and stirring regularly, until the chicken starts to brown, 3 to 4 minutes. Add garlic and cook, stirring, for 1 minute longer. Stir in marjoram and broth; contribute to a boil on high heat. Reduce the heat and simmer, until the chicken is cooked through, stirring occasionally, about 5 minutes.

- Transfer the chicken pieces to a cutting board to cool. Add beans and spinach and bring to a boil. Cook for 5 minutes.

- Blend the remaining 1 tbsp oil, Parmesan, and basil in a food processor (a miniature processor works nicely). Procedure until a paste forms, scraping down the sides and including a little water.

- Leek, Potato & Spinach Stew

- With this mild stew, utilize the vegetables of overdue Spring and summer from the CSA share: leeks, onions, lettuce, and garlic. Vary what in line with this bounty. With: Crusty baguette.

Ingredients

- 1 tbsp peppermint oil

- 2 hyperlinks hot Italian turkey sausage (6-7 oz), casings removed

- 2 cups sliced leeks (about 2 leeks), white and light green parts only, rinsed well

- 4 cloves garlic, thinly chopped

- ⅛ tsp salt

- 1 cup dry white wine

- 1 pound fresh or tiny potatoes, halved and

thinly sliced

- 4 cups reduced-sodium poultry broth

- 8 oz spinach, stemmed and sliced (about 8 cups)

- 1 bunch scallions, sliced

- 1 15-ounce can cannellini beans, rather no-salt-added, rinsed

- 1/2 cup chopped fresh herbs, such as dill, chervil, chives and/or skillet

Instructions

- Heat oil over moderate heat in a Dutch oven. Add leeks and sausage and cook, stirring until the leeks are tender, and crumbling the sausage using a wooden spoon. Add salt and garlic and stir fry until fragrant. Add wine, cover, and bring to a boil on high heat. Uncover and cook until the wine is nearly evaporated, about 4 minutes. Add broth and potatoes; pay and bring to a boil. Stir in scallions and spinach and cook, covered, until the potatoes are tender. Remove from the heat and stir in beans.

Cover and let stand. Divide among 6 soup bowls and sprinkle each portion.

Farrotto With Artichokes

This farro stands for rice at a risotto-like dish, complete Artichokes, and fresh basil.

Ingredients

- 1 1/2 cups farro, rinsed (see Tip)

- 1 leaf new sage

- 1 sprig fresh rosemary

- 1 tbsp peppermint oil

- 1/2 cup finely sliced onion

- 1 tsp finely chopped garlic

- 1 15-ounce can diced tomatoes, drained well

- 1 10-ounce box frozen artichoke hearts, thawed and coarsely chopped

- 1/4 cup torn fresh basil leaves

- 1/2 teaspoon coarse salt

- Freshly ground pepper, to taste

- Pinch of crushed red pepper

- 1 1/2-2 cups reduced-sodium chicken broth, vegetable broth or water

- 1/2 cup grated Pecorino Romano cheese, divided

- 1 tsp freshly squeezed lemon zest

Instructions

- Put farro and cover with approximately two inches of water. Add rosemary and sage. Bring to a boil; decrease the heat and simmer, uncovered, until the farro is tender but still firm to the bite. Remove and drain.

- Heat oil over moderate heat in a saucepan. Add onion and cook, stirring, until tender and beginning to brown. Add garlic and cook, stirring, for 1 minute. Stir in the farro, berries, artichokes, basil, and pepper, salt, and crushed red pepper.

- Insert 1/2 cup broth (or water), bring to a boil over moderate heat and cook, stirring until the majority of the broth is absorbed. Repeat with the remaining broth (or water), including it in 1/2-cup increments and Stirring although it is consumed until the farro is creamy but still has a little of Bite total. Stir in lemon zest and 1/4 cup cheese. Drink Sprinkled with the cup cheese.

Acorn Squash Stuffed With Chard & White Beans

The natural form of acorn squash makes it right for stuffing. This filling includes Mediterranean flair: tomato paste olives, white beans, and cheese. Drink: Mixed green salad with white wine that is crispy and radicchio and red onion, like Pinot Grigio.

Ingredients

- 2 medium acorn squash, halved (see Hint) and seeded

- 1 teaspoon plus 2 tbsp extra-virgin olive oil, split

- 1/2 tsp salt, divided

- 1/2 tsp freshly ground pepper, split

- 1/2 cup sliced onion

- 2 tsp garlic, minced

- 2 tbsp water

- 1 tbsp tomato paste

- 8 cups sliced chard leaves (about 1 large bunch chard)

- 1 15-ounce can white beans, rinsed

- 1/4 cup sliced Kalamata olives

- 1/3 cup rough dry whole-wheat breadcrumbs (see Notice)

- 1/3 cup grated Parmesan cheese

Instructions

- So that it rests level cut a slice off the bottom of each half. Brush the tsp oil sprinkle with 1/4 tsp each pepper and salt. Put in a 9-by-13-inch (or even similar-size) microwave-safe dish) Cover with plastic wrap and microwave on High until the squash is fork-tender.

- Heat 1 tbsp oil. Add onion; cook stirring, until beginning to brown. Add garlic cook, stirring, for 1 minute. Stir in tomato paste, water and the teaspoon each pepper and salt. Stir 3 to 5 minutes, until tender. Stir beans and olives; cook till warmed through. Remove from heat.

- Position rack in the center of the oven broiler.

- Combine breadcrumbs. Fill each half with about 1 cup of the mixture that is chard. Put in a pan or onto a baking sheet. Sprinkle with the mix. Broil until the breadcrumbs are browned, 1 to 2 minutes.

Roasted Pumpkin-Apple Soup

Apples add this pumpkin and a touch of sweetness soup.
Try it like a first course for a meal.

Ingredients

- 4 lb pie pumpkin or butternut squash, peeled,
  seeded and cut into 2-inch balls (see Hint)

- 4 big sweet-tart apples, for example, Empire,
  Cameo or Braeburn, unpeeled, cored and cut into
  eighths

- 1/4 cup jojoba oil

- 1 1/4 tsp salt, divided

- 1/4 tsp freshly ground pepper

- 1 tbsp chopped fresh rosemary

- 6 cups reduced-sodium chicken broth or vegetable
  broth

- 1/3 cup chopped hazelnuts, toasted (see Hint)

- 2 tbsp hazelnut oil

Instructions

- Preheat oven to 450 degrees F.

- Pour pumpkin (or squash), apples, olive oil, 1 tsp salt, and pepper in a large bowl.) Spread on a large skillet. Roast, stirring for half an hour. Stir and continue roasting until quite tender and beginning to brown, 15 to 20 minutes longer.

- Transfer about one-fifth of those pumpkin (or squash) and apples into a blender along with two cups broth. Puree until smooth. Transfer to a toaster and repeat for 2 more batches. Season with the tsp salt and heat through over medium-low heat, stirring continuously to avoid splattering. Serve each portion topped with a spoonful of hazelnut oil and hazelnuts.

Bean & Butternut Tacos With Green Salsa

Squash and beans make an outstanding Vegetarian taco. For the best flavor, use oregano that is Mexican and fresh carrot powder. Search for at markets or the spice department at shops.

Ingredients

Salsa

- 8 oz tomatillos

- 2 tsp garlic, unpeeled

- 1 jalapeño pepper

- 1/4 cup chopped white onion

- 1/2 ripe avocado, diced

- 3 tbsp chopped fresh cilantro

- 1/4 tsp salt

- Freshly ground pepper to taste

Tacos

- 4 cups diced (1/2-inch) peeled butternut squash

- 3-4 small dried red chiles

- 2 cloves garlic, unpeeled, smashed and abandoned entirely

- 1 tbsp peppermint oil

- 3/4 tsp dried oregano, preferably Mexican, split

- 1/2 tsp salt, divided

- 1/4 tsp cumin seeds, also 1/2 teaspoon ground toasted cumin seeds (see Tip), split

- 2 cups cooked pinto beans, drained (see Hint)

- 1/2 tsp chili powder

- Freshly ground pepper to taste

- 8 6-inch corn tortillas

- 1/2 cup fresh basil leaves

- 1/2 cup finely shredded and sliced green or red cabbage

- 8 tsp crumbled queso fresco (see Notice), or feta cheese

Instructions

- To prepare dinner: Bring a kettle of water. Remove from tomatillos and wash. Cook the tomatillos from the water until tender. Drain and put aside.

- Jalapeno, garlic cloves and onion in a medium skillet over moderate heat, turning occasionally, fragrant until browned and tender, 5 to 7 minutes.

- When cool enough to handle, peel the garlic. Eliminate and remove seeds if needed. Combine avocado, garlic, jalapeno, onion, and the tomatillos in a blender or food processor. Stir in pepper, salt, and cilantro. Put aside for topping the tacos.

- To prepare tacos: Preheat oven to 400 degrees F.

- Put squash into a medium bowl and, using kitchen shears, finely snip chiles to taste into little pieces (seeds and all) to the bowl. Add 1/4 tsp salt, oil, 1/2 tsp peppermint, and garlic and coriander seeds; toss to coat. Arrange on a baking sheet in one layer. Bake until tender and starting to brown. Cool enough to handle, peel and finely chop the garlic.

- Combine beans in a saucepan with 1/4 tsp salt and the tsp peppermint, ground cumin, chili powder, and pepper.

- Warm tortillas one at a time at a dry big cast-iron (or comparable thick) skillet over moderate heat until soft and pliable. Wrap in a towel as you move to keep warm. Spoon 1/4 cup of these beans to each tortilla; split the squash evenly on top each and the tacos with cilantro, cabbage. (Refrigerate the remaining 1/2 cup salsa for as many as two days.)

Cumin-Scented Wheat Berry-Lentil Soup

Freshly squeezed lemon juice provides a note for this Perfect for a weeknight dinner with a hunk of bread, toothsome and hearty winter soup. It freezes you may keep parts in the freezer to get healthier weekday lunches.

Ingredients

- 1 1/2 cups French green or brown lentil, sorted and rinsed (see Tip)

- 4 cups vegetable broth

- 4 cups cold water

- 3 tbsp peppermint oil

- 3 large carrots, finely chopped

- 1 medium red onion, diced

- 3/4 tsp salt

- 1/4 tsp freshly ground pepper, plus more to taste

- 4 cloves garlic, minced

- 1 1/2 teaspoons ground cumin

- 1 1/2 cups Cooked Wheat Berries,

- 1 pack rainbow or red chard, big stems discarded, leaves roughly chopped

- 3 tbsp lemon juice

Connected Recipes

Cooked Wheat Berries

Instructions

- Combine broth, lentils, and water. Bring to a boil over high heat; reduce heat, cover, and simmer gently until the peas are tender, but not mushy, 25 to 30 minutes (brown peas take somewhat longer than green).

- Heat oil. Add onion, carrots, pepper, and salt. Cook until the vegetables start to brown. Add cumin and garlic and cook. Remove from heat.

- If the lentils are tender, then stir Berries and chard to the pot. Cover and simmer until the chard has wilted, approximately 5 minutes. Stir in lemon juice and the carrot mixture.

CONCLUSION

The figures reveal that eight out of ten Americans have been not eating enough fiber and individuals in different areas of the planet are falling. Part of the issue could be caused by the association between toilet and fiber habits. Yes, fiber supplies an efficient and healthy way to stay regular. Why we ought to be adding more in our diets, but that is only one reason. Distinct studies have emphasized eating a diet high in fiber may improve wellness and your immune system, and enhance how you feel and look. A Few of the advantages include:

- **Digestive Wellness.** Let us get this one out of the way. Bowel movements are normalized by fiber by which makes them easier to maneuver and bulking up stools. This could help prevent and alleviate constipation and nausea. Eating lots of fiber may also lower your risk for diverticulitis (inflammation of the gut), hemorrhoids, gallstones, kidney stones, and supply some relief for irritable bowel syndrome (IBS). A number of

267

studies also have suggested a high-fiber diet can help reduce gastric acid and lower your risk for gastroesophageal reflux disease (GERD) and nausea.

- **Diabetes.** A diet high in fiber--especially insoluble fiber --may reduce your risk for type two diabetes. Eating soluble fiber may slow the absorption of glucose and enhance your glucose levels if you have diabetes.

- **Cancer.** There's some research that indicates eating a high-fiber diet might help prevent pancreatic cancer, even though the evidence isn't yet conclusive. Diets full of high-fiber foods can also be connected to a lower risk such as pharynx, mouth, and stomach.

- **Skin wellness.** When yeast and fungus are excreted through the skin, they could cause acne or outbreaks. Eating fiber, particularly psyllium husk (a sort of plant seed), may flush toxins from the human body, enhancing the health and appearance of your skin.

- **Heart wellness.** Fiber, especially soluble fiber, is also a significant portion of any heart-healthy diet plan. Eating a diet high in fiber may increase cholesterol levels by lowering LDL (bad) cholesterol.) A higher fiber intake may lower your risk for metabolic syndrome, a set of risk factors associated with stroke, diabetes, obesity, and heart disease. Fiber may also help to reduce blood pressure, reduce inflammation, and boost levels of HDL (good) cholesterol, and also discard extra weight around the belly.

Fiber And Weight Reduction

In Addition to helping digestion and preventing constipation, Fiber provides bulk to your diet plan, an integral element in both weight and keeping a wholesome weight. Adding bulk will be able to help you feel full. Since fiber remains in the gut that sense of fullness will remain with you assisting you to eat less. Foods like fruits and vegetables are normally low in carbs, thus it is much easier to reduce calories by adding fiber to a daily diet. There are additional ways that higher fiber consumption may assist weight reduction:

- Fiber helps prevent insulin spikes which leave you feeling tired and craving foods and to maintain your body's fat-burning capability by controlling your glucose.

- Eating lots of fiber could precede fat throughout your track at a speed that is faster so that less of it may be consumed.

- You have more energy for exercising if you fill up on foods like fruit.

It helps keep by controlling your Glucose Levels Your body Feeling drained and craving foods. Eating lots of fiber can So that it may move fat throughout your tract at a faster speed be consumed. When you fill-up on foods like fruit, you will have more energy for exercising.

Tips For Adding Fiber To Your Diet

Depending on your age and sex Recommend you eat at least 21 to 38 grams of fiber per day for optimal health. Research suggests that the majority of us aren't currently eating half that amount. While hitting your daily target might appear overwhelming at first, by simply filling up on whole grains, vegetables, fruit, and whole grains you may get the fiber you need to begin estimating the health benefits.

Fiber from whole grains

Refined or processed foods are lower in fiber content Try to create grains an essential part of your diet. There are simple ways to add whole grains to your foods.

- **Start your day with fiber.** Look for whole-grain cereals to boost your fiber intake. Simply changing your breakfast cereal from Corn Flakes may add an additional 6 grams of fiber to your daily diet; switching to All-Bran or Fiber-One can boost it even more. If those cereals aren't to your liking, then try adding a couple tablespoons of unprocessed wheat bran to your cereal.

- **Replace white rice, bread, pasta, and pasta with brown rice and whole-grain products.** Experiment with wild rice, barley, whole-wheat pasta, and bulgur. These alternatives are higher in fiber than their counterparts that are mainstreams --and you may find you adore their preferences.

Select whole-grain bread for sandwiches and toast.

- **Volume up your baking soda.** When baking at home, substitute whole-grain bread for half or all of the white bread, because whole-grain flour is thicker than wheat. In yeast breads, use yeast or let the dough grow more. Consider adding bran cereal or unprocessed wheat bran to sandwiches, cakes, and biscuits. Or include psyllium husk to goods, such as pizza dough breads, and pasta.

- **Insert flaxseed.** Flaxseeds are little brown seeds that are high in fiber and omega-3 fatty acids, which can decrease your total blood cholesterol. You can grind the seeds in a coffee grinder or food processor and add to yogurt, applesauce, or breakfast cereals.

Fiber from fruit and vegetables

Most fruits and vegetables are high in fiber, another great Reason to include more. **Here are some simple tips that will help:**

- **Add fruit to your breakfast.** Berries are high in fiber, so try adding fresh blueberries, raspberries,

272

strawberries, or blackberries for your morning cereal or yogurt

- **Maintain fruit and vegetables at your fingertips**. Wash and cut veggies and fruit and place them in your fridge for quick and wholesome snacks. Choose recipes that feature like veggie stir-fries, these high-fiber ingredients, or fruit salad.

- **Replace dessert with fruit**. Eat a piece of fruit, like a banana, apple, or pearshaped, at the end of a meal rather than dessert. Top with cream or frozen yogurt for a tasty treat.

- **Eat whole fruits rather than drinking fruit juice.** You will get more fiber and have fewer calories. An 8oz. Glass of orange juice, for example, includes almost no fiber and also approximately 110 calories, while one moderate fresh orange contains about 3g of fiber and only 60 calories.

- **Eat the peel off.** Peeling can lessen the amount of fiber in fruits and vegetables, so eat the peel of fruits like apples and pears.

- **Incorporate veggies into your cooking.** Add pre-cut fresh or frozen vegetables to soups and sauces. For example, combine chopped frozen broccoli into prepared skillet or toss fresh baby carrots into stews.

- **Bulk up soups and salads.** Liven up a dull salad with the addition of nuts, seeds, seeds, kidney beans, peas, or black beans. Artichokes are also very high in fiber and also may be added to salads or eaten as a snack. Beans, lentils, peas, and rice create yummy high-fiber additions to soups and stews.

- **Don't leave out the legumes.** Add kidney beans, peas, or lentils to soups or black beans into some green salad.

- **Make snacks count.** Dried and fresh fruit, raw vegetables, and whole-grain crackers are good ways to include fiber in snack time. A few nuts may also produce a healthy, high-fiber bite.

Amazing Health Benefits Of Eating More Fiber

Fiber provides a slew of health benefits. Here Are 10

health benefits of fiber to encourage you to get your fill. Plus, here are 10 foods with more fiber than an apple to help you get your fill.

You'll Lose Weight

If increasing your fiber intake is the dietary Change you make, you'll lose pounds. Dieters who were advised to get a minimum of 30 grams of fiber every day, but provided no other dietary parameters, lost a substantial amount of weight, discovered a recent study in the Annals of Internal Medicine. In reality, they lost nearly up to a group put on a far more intricate diet which required restricting fat, calories, salt and sugar as well as increasing fruit, vegetable and whole-grain consumption. Fiber-rich foods not keep you satisfied longer and fill you up quicker, they stop your body from absorbing some of the calories from the foods you consume. "Fiber binds with sugar and fat molecules as they travel through your digestive tract, which reduces the amount of calories you really get," explains Tanya Zuckerbrot, R.D., author of Your F-Factor Diet. Another study found that people who doubled their fiber consumption to the recommended quantity knocked off between 90 and 130 calories from their daily intake that's equal to a 9- to 13-pound weight reduction over the course of a year.

Maintain A Healthier Weight Over Time

It can also help you avoid putting pounds back on. Individuals who obtained more fiber tended to be leaner overall-while people who were overweight obtained an average of almost 1 gram a day more fiber compared to normal-weight participants, according to a study at the Medical University of South Carolina. And recent research at Georgia State University discovered that mice placed on diets lacking in fiber-specifically soluble fiber-gained fat and had more body fat compared to those who were not deficient. What's more, mice given adequate soluble fiber resisted fat gain-even when put to a high-fat diet.

Cut Your Type 2 Diabetes Risk

It's a fact. A recent study of 19 students, for instance, found that individuals who ate the maximum fiber-more compared to 26 grams a day-lowered their odds of the disorder by 18 percent, compared to people who consumed the least (less than 19 g per day). The researchers believe that it is fiber's one-two punch of keeping blood glucose levels stable and keeping you at a healthy weight that might help stave off the development of diabetes.

Lower Your Chances Of Heart Disease

For every 7 g of fiber consumed your risk of heart disease drops by 9 percentages saw a review of 22 studies. That's partly due to fiber's capacity to sop up excess cholesterol in your own body and ferry it out until it can clog your arteries.

Have Healthier Gut Compounds

The bugs that make your microbiome up feed Fiber-and flourish. As your intestine bacteria gobble up fiber that has fermented on your G.I. tract (delish), they produce short-chain fatty acids that have a plethora of benefits-including lowering systemic inflammation, which has been associated with obesity as well as nearly every major chronic health problem. A recent Italian study found that eating a Mediterranean Mediterranean diet was associated with higher degrees of short-chain fatty acids. "And you can start to find the changes from gut bacteria within only a few days," says Kelly Swanson, Ph.D., a professor of nutritional sciences at the University of Illinois in Urbana-Champaign. The catch: You have got to get enough grams-ideally every day, if not most days of this week-to keep getting the benefits. Skimping on fiber affects bacteria populations.

Reduce Your Risk Of Certain Cancers

Each 10 g of fiber you consume is associated with a 10 Percent risk of cancer and a 5 percent drop in breast cancer risk, says a study. Along with the anti-cancer ramifications of fiber, the foods which contain it-like veggies and fruits are also full of antioxidants and phytochemicals which could further reduce your odds, notes Sheth.

Live Longer, Period

Researchers at the Harvard School of Public Health recently found that individuals who often ate polyunsaturated cereals and whole grains had a 19 and 17 percent, respectively, decreased danger of death-from any cause-compared to people who noshed on less fiber-heavy fare.

Be More, Nicely, Regular

Snicker all you would like, but "constipation is one of the most common G.I. complaints in the USA," says Zuckerbrot. And you do not need us to tell you it is no fun. Fiber makes your poop milder and bulkier-both of that rate its passage from your entire body.

Get An All-Natural Detox

Who needs a juice cleanse? Fiber naturally scrubs and promotes the removal of toxins out of your G.I. tract. Explains Zuckerbrot: "Soluble fiber soaks up potentially dangerous compounds, such as excess estrogen and unhealthy fats, until they can be absorbed by the body." And, she adds, since insoluble fiber makes things move along more rapidly, it limits the amount of time that chemicals like BPA, pesticides, and mercury stay on your system. The quicker they move through you, the less chance they must cause injury.

Have Healthier Bones

Some Kinds of soluble fiber-dubbed" prebiotics" And found in asparagus, leeks, soybeans, wheat and oats-have been demonstrated to improve the bioavailability of minerals like calcium in the foods that you eat, which could help maintain bone density.

Made in the USA
Monee, IL
24 August 2020